A SINGULAR VIEW

Michael O. Hughes
Publisher/Editor
307 B, Maple Avenue West
Vienna, Virginia 22180-4307 USA
www.asingularview.com

Seventh U.S. Edition, 2009, Printed in Canada
Spanish Edition, 2008

Copyright © 1972 (First Edition), 1978 (Second Printing), 1979 (Revised Printing), 1985, 1994, 2004 (Revised 6th Edition), 2006 (Revised 7th Edition), 2007, 2008.

Library of Congress Cataloging in Publication Data;
Brady, Frank B.
A Singular View; The Art of Seeing With One Eye
Revised 7th U.S. Edition, 2008
ISBN 10: 0-9614639-2-9
ISBN 13: 978-0-961463-92-2

Illustrations by Juan García and Craig Luce; certified medical illustrators

Originally published in 1972 by Medical Economics Company, A Litton Industries Division, at Oradell, NJ 07649. ISBN 0-87489-224-4

A SINGULAR VIEW

THE ART OF SEEING WITH ONE EYE

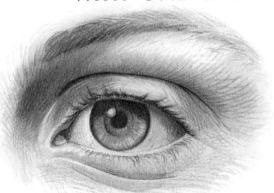

FRANK B. BRADY

Contents

Using This Book

One thing about books on techniques of any kind is that some of the tips will only sink in after some time, so plan on rereading this book in several weeks or a month. Then you can evaluate your progress and be certain to get the most from it in review.

You've probably noticed that this book is printed in larger type than usual. Although a normal single eye will have no more of a problem coping with even fine print than a pair of good eyes, the larger print here is because some readers may be recovering from a recent eye loss or other vision problems.

A variety of useful things and further tips for the newly monocular is reviewed and linked to the Internet site **www.asingularview.com**. Most public and school libraries now offer access to the Internet free of charge, so make use of it. Your access code is numbered on the back page of this book.

I hope that this will be helpful to you. Your world awaits!

Losing the Sight of an Eye: You Are Not Alone

"The eye is the window to the soul." While this is more than only poetically true, there is an aura around the eye that makes its loss seem all the more tragic. While this book is striving to lay aside your fears about what your new world holds for you, we should take a moment to recognize that this loss of vision, this loss of the use of a precious organ, this—your loss—is often accompanied by depression and despair.

Yes, you have another. Yes, we will work together to aid in your recovery. Yes, you can have a very full and happy life! But the loss of this one thing is loaded with emotion. Many resources can help you deal with this emotional loss—it has happened to us, too.

Some of the people you will meet in this book have made huge strides to cope with this themselves. Others have not even slowed down to own their grief. But all have a shared experience and can help you find your feet in recovering your life.

Certainly, counselors of several kinds have been or will be presented to you. You may have wanted to ignore them, wanted to ignore your pain. You may have felt ashamed or lessened, even judged by this occurrence. Only you can decide how best to deal with this— just know that there is a variety of emotional help available and solutions to everyday fears. Only you have to reach out.

There is no other symbol of our humanity more revered than the human eye. It has been thought to have powers that it cannot deserve—it is, after all, only an eye. But this is *your* eye. Perhaps yours was born that way and never saw light, or, alternatively, it was taken in an instant—or anything in-between.

Annie N. wrote, "There are some days when I look in the mirror and find myself in tears. 'Why,' I wondered, 'did this happen

to *me?*'" Seek these answers with your family and loved ones—
and remember there are professionals who can help, too.

Perhaps you think that no one else can understand. There are
many who have lived through this—over 50,000 in North
America alone!

We will go through this process one chapter at a time, so you
understand that life goes on, and how, and why things are different. I just wanted to let you know that you are not alone.

Frank B. Brady

Dedication

This book is dedicated to my father, Ben, and to all who have demonstrated a remarkable resiliency of the human spirit by transmuting their experience of physical and emotional trauma to embrace life more deeply and joyously.

—*Michael O. Hughes*
Publisher/Editor, A Singular View

Introduction

by Julius Axelrod, Nobel Laureate

At the age of 21 when I was working in the Department of Bacteriology at New York University Medical School, I lost the sight in my left eye through a laboratory accident there.

While I continued my studies and a very active life, I wish this book had been available to me at the time it happened. It would have saved me much time in adjusting to monocular vision.

Overall, losing the vision in one eye has not been a real handicap in my life. My career has required constant use of my eyes for measuring chemicals, using a microscope and other complex instruments, and reading an immense amount of scientific literature. All of my work has included experiments that demand care, skill and precision.

For many years, I wore a black patch; like the Hathaway Man, this made me look like a dashing figure. Due to further medical reasons, my left eye was removed about thirteen years ago, and I had an artificial eye made near my home in Vienna, Virginia.

Frank Brady's book, *A Singular View,* pointed out various things that I was unaware of, even being monocular myself. I was happy to find it, even years after my own recovery. This book would have made my recovery quicker and more complete.

In the ways of science, we accept that the outcome of an experiment is uncertain until proven upon review. This little book contains suggestions and tips that have been tested and collected in an easily accessible format available to everyone.

I fully endorse Frank Brady's efforts. His purpose here and its effects are evident in the lives of several persons of my personal knowledge, and it has helped me as well. This small book should be available to anyone wishing to guide their own life or help a loved one regain the activities of daily life as they experienced them before.

While the large print edition was offered early in its publishing history, this new edition is full of illustrations that allow access to the information even by patients with further reading problems. In a practical way, Frank has made recovery shorter and more complete for those with this affliction, whatever their socio-economic situation. I applaud his efforts in writing this book and look forward to its reaching a worldwide audience.

At age 90, I still drive to my laboratory and carry on an active life.

—Julius Axelrod, Ph.D.
Bethesda, Maryland
2003

Editorial Note:

Dr. Julius Axelrod received the Nobel Prize in 1970 for his work in brain chemistry and drugs that affect the heart and mind. His work in identifying the mechanism of action of a new compound, acetaminophen, resulted in such brand names as Tylenol. This work was even before his Ph.D. dissertation from George Washington University. As he continued his work at the National Institutes of Health, he identified drug-metabolizing enzymes in the liver. Further, he revealed the re-uptake mechanism of neurotransmitters in the synapse, thus demonstrating the action of cocaine and certain antidepressants. He has enjoyed a long teaching career and remains Scientist Emeritus there.

From the Foreword to the First Edition

When Frank Brady told me that he was toying with the idea of writing "a sort of manual for the newly one-eyed," my response was instant and positive. "This is a book that should be written," I told him, "and you're the one to do it."

He has made a huge contribution to the recovery of nearly 50,000 annual newcomers to this condition.

I think this book will also interest anyone who is curious about the workings of one of nature's most fabulous creations—the human eye. And it will certainly captivate every person who enjoys reading about the human capacity for adaptation.

—John W. McTigue, M.D.
Ophthalmologist

From the Preface to the First Edition

Eyes are mankind's closest bond to the environment, and any threat to vision is certain to produce massive anxieties. Even the loss of one eye can be a matter of enormous concern to an active individual in love with living. Will one ever be able to work again, to dive, to fly, to win a mate, even to make it across the street?

I went through all these anxieties when I lost my good right eye. The experiences I went through brought home that there was very little guidance available. The techniques I used to become accustomed to being one-eyed were learned the hard way. Some seemed appropriate to the several others I was asked to help.

Slowly a notion of a book formed, and I hope that this book will spare you some of the bumps and bruises I earned while trying to figure things out on my own.

—Frank Brady

Acknowledgments

One of the most pleasant surprises connected with the preparation of this book has been the enthusiastic response to almost any request for assistance. While this list is incomplete, I must thank a few who have been especially generous with their resources.

Aileen, Neill and Elizabeth
Lou Brady
The American Medical Association's Committee on
    Medical Aspects of Automotive Safety
The Federal Aviation Administration,
    Office of Aviation Medicine
The American Association of Motor Vehicle Administrators
American Academy of Opthalmology
American Anaplastology Association
American Optometric Association
American Society of Ocularists
Bethesda Naval Hospital
Prevent Blindness America
United States Department of Veterans Affairs
Dr. Michael Berenhaus, Optometrist
Dr. Robert Allen, Ophthalmologist
Dr. William Bearden, Ophthalmologist
Dr. Ken Blaylock, Ophthalmologist
Dr. Bruce Carter, Ophthalmologist
Dr. Brian Conway, Ophthalmologist
Dr. Albert Cytryn, Ophtalmologist
Dr. William Deegan, Ophthalmologist
Dr. Paul Gavaris, Ophthalmologist
Dr. Todd Goodglick, Ophthalmologist
Dr. Michael Grant, Ophthalmologist
Dr. Kurt Guelzow, Ophthalmologist

Dr. Nicholas Iliff, Ophthalmologist
Dr. Sara Kaltreider, Ophthalmologist
Dr. Tim Malone, Ophthalmologist
Dr. Shannath Merbs, Ophthalmologist
Dr. Stephen Newman, Ophthalmologist
Dr. Narieman Nik, Ophthalmologist
Dr. Kevin Perman, Ophthalmologist
Dr. Arthur Perry, Ophthalmologist
Dr. Polly Purgason, Ophthalmologist
Dr. Soheila Rostami, Ophthalmologist
Dr. George Sandborn, Ophthalmologist
Dr. Kevin Scott, Ophthalmologist
Dr. Carol Shields, Ophthalmologist
Dr. Jerry Shields, Ophthalmologist
Dr. Marc Shields, Ophthalmologist
Dr. Jeff Zuravleff, Ophthalmologist
Wills Eye Hospital, Philadelphia
Wilmer Eye Clinic, Baltimore
University of Iowa, Department of Ophthalmology
University of Michigan, Department of Ophthalmology
University of Virginia, Department of Ophthalmology
Annie and Nan Nelson
Institute for Families
Pennsylvania College of Optometry
Julius Axelrod, Ph.D., Nobel Laureate

Dr. John W. McTigue, without whose encouragement, prodding and generous assistance this book might not have gotten past the procrastination stage.

We wish to thank the literally hundreds of persons who have written with suggestions, ideas and encouragement. They have convinced us that this book has fulfilled many of our original goals.

Chapter 1

An Unhappy Landing

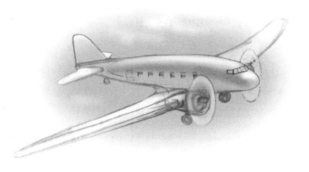

I HAVE NO memory of being hit. I only recall a dazed awareness that something was wrong, very wrong . . . that the pilot was swinging our plane into position for a landing . . . asking the tower for runway lights . . . calling for an ambulance to meet the plane.

Then Tom Wright, the third man aboard, was helping me out of the cockpit, where I had been flying co-pilot, and onto the couch so that he could take my place and assist in the landing.

Seemingly countless minutes later (actually less than three), I was being lifted into the ambulance. Exactly seven minutes after the accident, I was getting skilled emergency treatment in an Air Force hospital.

Our plane, a research DC-3, had been on the last leg of a flight from Chicago via Washington that April evening. We'd been skimming over Long Island after sunset and were preparing to land at Grumman Field when the craft was struck. Captain Macatee (who would later fly the first scheduled jetliner across America) had no idea what had hit us until after the landing, when he found a five-pound mallard duck in the cockpit.

The big bird, one of a migrating pair that had collided with us, had crashed through the windshield at over 200 miles per hour and struck me full in the face, bouncing my head against the aluminum bulkhead behind me. A large dent in the heavy metal attested to the force of the blow. Later, when I had a chance to examine it, I realized that the bulkhead had actually kept my neck from snapping.

In my work in aviation safety, I had recently taken a keen interest in a procedure to test the resistance of cockpit windshields to just such bird strikes. The method was to fire a newly killed chicken from an air-cannon at various test mockups.

The test results have made windshields in aircraft of all types safer—from private props to fighter jets—and stronger windshields had been ordered for our DC-3. They arrived shortly after my accident.

This testing method is still used today, firing chickens at up to 700 miles per hour—very similar to the way mockups of the space shuttle *Columbia* were tested to see if ice had injured the wing on launch. This air-cannon method was subsequently used by engineers in other countries using frozen birds—only the windshields were being utterly destroyed every time. When they asked how our results were so much better, we faxed them back, "Thaw the chickens first!"

Chapter 2

An Awkward Take-Off

IT WAS SEVERAL days before the doctors decided that I was strong enough to hear the bad news: My right eye had been damaged beyond repair. It would have to be removed without further delay, they told me, in order to prevent a sympathetic reaction from developing in the good remaining eye.

The verdict didn't really surprise me, even though the damaged eye had been kept under wraps all this time. And there was really no point in brooding about it. I began instead to develop an overwhelming curiosity about the future. Would my world be changed when viewed through a single eye? Would my activities be restricted? Would I ever drive a car again? Fly a plane? Play golf or even just cross a street with a reasonable expectation of reaching the other side alive?

In the course of my life I'd met quite a few people who had lost the vision of one eye. Now I spent long hours in my hospital bed, anxiously trying to recall all the details I'd learned about them so I could apply this knowledge to my own circumstances.

There was Bob, for instance, who wore a patch on one eye and delighted in driving his car at 90 miles an hour on winding rural roads. I had no desire to duplicate Bob's madness, but was encouraged to think that the loss of half his vision had restrained him no more than the laws of the land!

On the other hand, I knew that Bob had lost his eye at a very early age, and wondered if this might be the key to his amazing adaptation. I was already past 30. Would I be able to regain enough of my old skills—to say nothing of acquiring some necessary new ones—and continue the life I'd been leading?

My thoughts turned more hopefully to another acquaintance, one who had lost an eye when he was already a grown man. Cliff, a co-worker in an engineering lab, had won the respect of everyone for his impeccable craftsmanship. We had often discussed the techniques he used to gauge distances and manipulate instruments, information that would now be very useful to me.

Then there was the great Wiley Post, one of my boyhood heroes. With only one good eye to guide him, Post had twice circled the

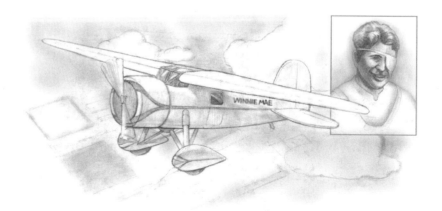

Wiley Post and his plane the Winnie Mae.

globe by air, aided only by the relatively crude instruments of the time. Pondering his long solo flights and his landings under the most difficult conditions enabled me to feel that the loss of one eye, while unfortunate, need not handicap me for the rest of my life.

I continued to search for reasons to be optimistic, even as I was confronted with more doubts. A hospital environment has a way of magnifying fears and misgivings to unrealistic proportions, especially at night. There were times when I felt agonizingly sure that neither my personal nor my professional life would ever be the same again.

On the day I was to be discharged, a pleasant young man came into my room and introduced himself as Dr. Drake.

"How are you doing?" he asked.

"Just fine," I answered truthfully. The prospect of finally getting back into action had buoyed my spirits.

Dr. Drake sat down and began what initially seemed like a casual, innocent conversation. As his questions became more penetrating, I realized that I was on the receiving end of a very skillful psychiatric evaluation. Its purpose was to discover if the battering of the whole right half of my face and the loss of an eye had thrown me into a state of depression.

Strangely enough, the effect of the interview raised my mood almost to the point of elation. I began to feel like the boy who, after surgery on his hands, asked his doctor, "Do you think I'll be able to play the piano now?"

"Definitely," said the doctor.

"Wow!" screamed he boy. "That's great! I never could play before!"

Apparently, I emerged from the interview with passing marks, for when Dr. Drake rose to leave, he wished me goodbye and good luck.

I reached to grasp his outstretched hand—and missed by a mile!

Chapter 3

Jolts of Reality

WHILE IT DIDN'T take me too long to master the art of hand shaking, the real world that was waiting to wake me up from my hospital daydreams had many more rude jolts in store for me.

Outside the hospital, I hailed a cab and stepped off the sidewalk as it approached. Underestimating the height of the curb, I jolted forward and nearly ended up under the taxi's wheels.

At a party in my honor, I volunteered to mix a martini for a thirsty young woman. I mixed it perfectly. Then, when she held up her glass to receive it, I poured it on the floor.

My "grand entrance" at another party became a spectacle. I descended the stairs, raised my hands in greeting to the guests, stepped into the living room and fell forward in amazement. The last step had disguised itself as part of the living room floor.

My first try at table tennis was a disaster that stirred my friends to a pitying quietness.

It seemed everybody in the world had suddenly decided to move in on my right (sightless) side, and I was in a constant state of collision with them.

At a restaurant our waitress was serving hot soup. She came up on my right side just as my hands were describing the size of a fish I'd once caught. I caught the soup bowl this time and received a painful burn that lingered on my right arm for several days—evidence of a newborn clumsiness.

For some time I was to live in a world of awkwardness and embarrassment, much of which I could have been spared if only someone had given me the explanations and helpful tips that appear in the following chapters.

It was perhaps with justifiable trepidation that, at the urging of friends, I got behind the wheel of a car two days after leaving the hospital. I tried to cling to the right lane, but found it hard to judge my distance from the parked cars. Terrors seemed to spill in from all directions at the intersections, but particularly from the right.

I had to swivel my head in much wider arcs, much faster and much more frequently than I ever had before, and I needed a heightened alertness to cope with each new danger. I was pathetically grateful for the "co-pilot" on my right during that first nightmarish ride through town.

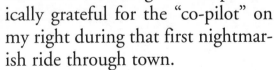

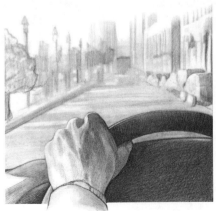

Out on the open highway, however, things went more smoothly, and some of my former ease at the wheel returned. I quickly learned to lag a little farther than usual behind vehicles and soon began to understand why my old friend Bob had no qualms about going 90 miles an hour once his path was cleared of traffic.

It was while driving at slow speeds, threading my way between other cars on the city street or backing into a parking space, that I experienced the most serious difficulty in judging distances. Nevertheless, I ended that first drive with certainty that this was one activity I wouldn't have to give up—at no time had I felt that I was driving in an unsafe manner. Any loss of visual perception was more than offset by the enforced—and often excruciating—increase in alertness.

Chapter 4

Flying High

THAT SAME HYPERAWARENESS sustained me as I tested myself in a variety of skills for which I had a well established "know-how," but a recently acquired uneasiness about my "do-how." For it was back in my boyhood that I had gathered the assortment of knacks and knowledge that later guided my choice of career.

At 16 I was a glider buff, obtaining my pilot's license in a craft that school chums and I had built and taught ourselves to fly. Soon after that I became fascinated by ham radios, building and operating amateur stations. As I grew up, I was drawn into the field of radio engineering. My old interest in flying, however, led me to aviation electronics, where I found a new specialty—the development of instrument approach and landing systems.

World War II created a demand for men with this type of background. As a young civilian engineer, I was soon in charge of a siz-

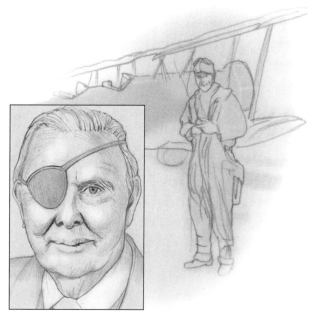

I flew long before my accident and long after!

able instrument landing program for the Allied Forces in Europe. After the war I joined the civil aviation industry to help the airlines adapt to peacetime use of the air traffic control and instrument landing systems that had proved so successful. It was in this capacity that I was directing a flight research program on the night of my accident.

Though my main interest had always been my work, I don't believe I neglected my social or outdoor activities. Swimming and sailing were my favorite sports, augmented by a bit of tennis and golf. After the loss of my eye, each of these old activities presented new challenges as I cautiously, problem by problem, worked out new ways of coping.

Shortly after the accident I was back at my job and having no difficulty filling it. The flight research program had been dropped, so I was no longer required to fly. I flew anyway—partly to find out how I'd do at it, and partly because it was in my blood.

In many ways I found it easier than driving. I had no trouble making the distance judgments that are required for landing and other maneuvers. And the hyperawareness that I've acquired since the accident easily compensates for the loss of side vision. In fact, I would go so far as to say that there has been a *net gain* in safety.

Perhaps my most demanding post-accident project was the building of a ship model to exact standards. It's true that threading all those tiny deadeyes, setting up the rigging at a scale of one-eighth inch to the foot, and doing all the other fine detailed work wasn't easy; the point is that it could be done—and done with no loss of quality in workmanship.

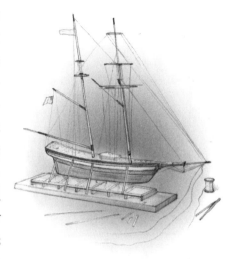

All in all my adaptation was going well at the end of the first year. By the end of two years, I was totally at ease in my normal activities, even though I was still undergoing plastic surgery for cosmetic reasons. Some jobs took a little extra time and effort, and many situations called for the heightened sense of awareness that I've already mentioned. But if I sometimes regarded my new condition as a damned nuisance, I never considered it a handicap—in my career, in my hobbies, or in my personal life.

It was toward the end of this rehabilitation period that, through a chance meeting, my personal life took a highly affirmative turn. The success of my adaptation was proved by the fact that for months I made weekly trips from Washington, through Maryland and Pennsylvania, driving seven hours at a stretch—often at night—to woo the future Mrs. Brady.

Chapter 5

How About You?

So MUCH FOR my story. Now what about yours? If you're reading this book, chances are that you or a loved one has recently lost the full use of one eye. Right now uncertainty rules your mind: "Will I be able to regain my life, schedule and activities?" Let's take a look at some of the factors that may help or hinder you on the road back.

Every person is right-eyed or left-eyed (just as one is right-handed or left-handed), depending on which half of the brain is dominant. The right hand, foot and eye are controlled by the left hemisphere of the brain, which in most persons is dominant. Likewise, the right hemisphere controls the left side of the body. Obviously, the loss of your favored or dominant hand would call for a far longer and more difficult readjustment than loss of the left; it would entail a massive re-education of the brain.

To a lesser degree, the same is true of the eyes. If your brain is used to receiving messages and making decisions on the basis of information received from your right eye, and that's the one you lost, the road back is going to be a bit more difficult for you. In my own case, it was the right, or favored, eye that was removed, so that was a hindrance to my recovery. We'll call the side that has the loss of sight the "affected side."

While eye dominance is perhaps the single most important factor in adapting, there are several other factors, such as *visual acuity* (or "sharpness of vision"—see the glossary at the back of this book). If the "working" eye has good vision (as in my case), it can more easily take over the duties of its lost mate, even though that mate may have been the favored one. If the good eye has poor vision and was also the secondary eye, then it's going to take more time and effort to adjust. You will adjust either way, of course, just more slowly.

Age is another important factor (the younger you are, the better). Another is the speed of the loss (gradual or sudden). If the one eye deteriorates over a long period of time, the good eye has a chance to accustom itself slowly to the increased workload and make an orderly transition.

Then, of course, a lot depends on how far you want or need to carry your adaptation. Some occupations (such as pilot or machinist) and some hobbies (such as racket sports or sewing) call for more accurate depth perception than is the average. Coping with this requires a longer and more determined effort than average, too. Still, the best thing for you to think now is that it *is* possible to regain most all of your earlier capacity and activities. I can prove it!

Each person's psychological reaction to the loss of an eye is different—ranging all the way from "What's the use of living?" to "I hardly notice the difference."

While I was still in the early stages of my own recovery, I got an urgent call one night from a friend, asking would I please talk with his 18-year-old nephew who had recently lost an eye as the result of a car accident. He said Fred had come home from the hospital in such a severe depression that his family was greatly concerned about what he might do, and didn't have a clue how to help him. Despondent, he sounded ready to do himself harm! Alarmed, I hastily agreed to visit Fred. Besides, it might also help me to reach out in this way.

It turned out that Fred and I had a lot more in common than the loss of an eye. He mumbled that he loved gliders, so we immediately spoke the same language. As soon as we got on that subject, he said that the cause of his despair was that he was certain he'd never be able to fly a glider again. I assured him from my own direct experience that he was completely mistaken. I excitedly told him about some of the tricks I'd learned to compensate while flying, and at last he was convinced—his mood changed quickly from one of self-destruction to an eagerness to get on with his recovery and back into the air. The next day his family's relief was obvious—Fred was smiling again!

But not all psychological reactions to the loss of an eye are so simple. Others feel they must overcompensate for the loss by learning to do more than they could before. The frustrations that can come with such unrealistic expectations can sometimes call for prolonged psychiatric help—and you would do well to seek this if depression continues. It is my sincere hope that the tips and tricks I will discuss here will help you know that there *are* solutions—and that a full and active life is a very real and available goal. Your success is limited only by your willingness to start studying the information in this book.

Often, well meaning friends and even professionals tend to minimize the loss of an eye. This is a very important part of the body that causes much grief and sadness when it is lost, notes Nancy Mansfield, Ph.D., Executive Director, Institute for Families (Director, Social Services) at Childrens Hospital, Los Angeles.

On the other hand, some people of great character and determination become even greater successes by overcompensating. For example, in the 1950s the great entertainer, Sammy Davis, Jr., was in a car accident that damaged his left eye beyond repair. While recuperating he vowed: "When I come back, there can be no 'He's almost as good as he ever was.' I've got to be better." And within four months he was back, working hard, this time right at the top of his profession. Nothing wrong with that!

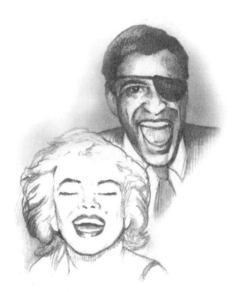

With only one eye, Sammy Davis, Jr. enjoyed a diverse career, which included working with Marilyn Monroe.

Chapter 6

Seeing in 3-D

IF YOU'VE ENJOYED fairly normal vision since birth, it may never have occurred to you that a great deal of what we call "seeing" is really a learned skill. We take it for granted that any creature born with eyes can "see". But show a dog a photograph of his beloved master, and he won't display any sign of recognition. Not only does it takes a trained brain to be able to see the likeness of a human face in the simple shapes and variations of color on a piece of paper, the human mind is the only brain on this planet that recognizes itself as a separate being. That is a learned and blessed ability.

I once witnessed the reaction of a young boy who was watching his father's plane take off from a private airfield. As the plane soared away into the blue, the child began to scream. "Daddy will be back soon," his mother reassured him. But that wasn't what was bothering the boy. "Look!" he screamed even louder, pointing to the tiny speck in the sky, "Daddy's getting small!"

The youngster's fear that his father was becoming impossibly small only confirmed what scientific studies have found—that the gift of sight doesn't necessarily give a person perception, or the ability to grasp the meaning of what is seen. This is learned.

Vision is the whole process, and it is made up of several parts. Vision requires 1) a stimulus of reflected light, 2) an organ to perceive the light (the eye), 3) an organ to interpret the light into images (the brain), and 4) another area of the brain to associate the images into known or unknown pictures and store the images into memory.

Persons who have been blind from birth, and then suddenly have eyesight granted to them by surgery or some other miracle, have a whole new language to learn. For instance, it takes some time before they can interpret a picture, just as it must have taken the little boy some time to learn to relate small size to distance. They are training and programming the brain to make sense of the world around them. In the same way, recovering from partial loss of the vision you've learned and have used all your life entails a whole new learning experience.

Some people who've always had normal vision try to make the transition from two eyes to one by letting nature take its course—by merely coping as circumstances present themselves. Such an unorganized approach will eventually get you there, yes—but by doing a bit of homework and reading this book, you can speed up this process and smooth it out, gain confidence, and avoid mishaps.

The first thing you need to understand is the nature of the change that has taken place. What is it, exactly, that you have lost? And what is it that you still have?

What's the Difference?

Visual Situation	One Eye vs. Two
Visual acuity	Small to no disadvantage
Visual field	Moderate disadvantage
Contrast	Equal or better with experience
Direct light	Equal
Diffuse light	Equal
Background light	Equal
Glare	Equal
Distance from task	Small to no disadvantage
3-D stereo vision	Significant disadvantage
Depth perception	Moderate to significant disadvantage

With many tasks, you will see about the same as before. Of course, if a wide visual field is needed for an activity, there will be some impairment for which you can compensate. As far as the distance to the task, or the lighting or glare in your environment, or contrast is involved, your decrease is hardly noticeable.

The only time there is a real difference is when 3-D vision is demanded of the task, and you are not in a position to move your head. So when might that happen? Well, for you, driving will be the largest issue, but that's manageable because you can still move your head and are usually already moving (see relative movement in glossary).

There may be some tasks that you actually perform better than your two-eyed colleagues, because you are more aware of *all* your tools. The binocular (two-eyed) population relies heavily on depth perception, less on contrast or other cues, you are becoming aware of now. Practice and time will make the difference.

THE WAY THE EYE WORKS

The human eye is certainly one of nature's most amazing creations. Just as humans stand at the top of the evolutionary pyramid, vision is the most highly developed of the human senses. Each eyeball is really like a wonderfully crafted miniature camera.

With a camera, the light enters through a lens, is focused onto a recording device (film or digital), recorded and stored. The human eye does the same thing.

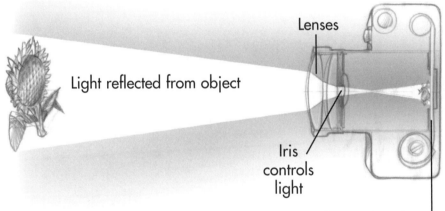

Lenses

Light reflected from object

Iris controls light

Film or digital recorder

When both these cameras are in good working order, one need only to open one's eyelids to obtain a continuous view of the world in glorious, dimensional, living color. We'll learn more about how the two eyes work together in the next chapter.

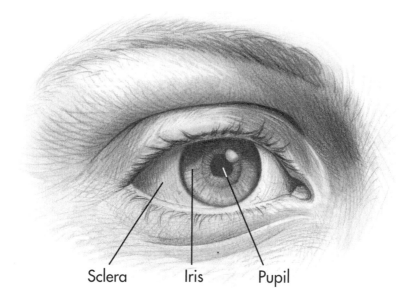

Sclera   Iris   Pupil

EYE ANATOMY

Any part of the environment of light that commands your attention, whether it be a mountaintop or the eye of a needle, first enters the eye through the cornea.

This tough, clear portion is part of the white sclera surrounding the entire eye—sort of like the case of the camera, housing and protecting the other working parts. The clear cornea is more than just a "window"—it also does most of the work to bend light into an image on the back of the eye.

Light then passes through the watery fluid behind the cornea to pass through the pupil, which is really just a hole in the colored iris. The iris is the blue, green or brown part that controls the amount of light entering by making the pupil larger or smaller. The pupil looks black because there's no light coming back out the hole.

The light then passes through the lens, which can fine-tune

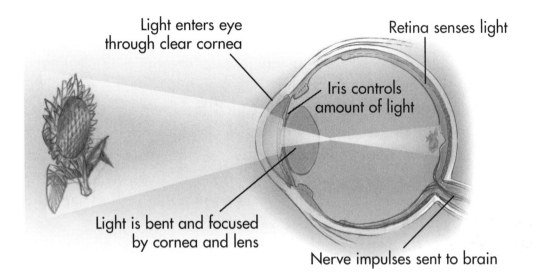

Light enters eye through clear cornea

Retina senses light

Iris controls amount of light

Light is bent and focused by cornea and lens

Nerve impulses sent to brain

the focus whether objects are closer or nearer to us. The light gets more focused as it travels through the vitreous body to the retina, which acts as the film (or digital pixels) to receive the light. The tissue-thin retina breaks the image into nerve impulses, which it transmits to the brain through the optic nerve.

It's the brain that makes these impulses into a picture—all the way back in the occipital lobe, which sends the image to associative areas in the brain so that we understand the picture and store it as a memory.

This brain part is usually still working just fine for you and me— but to see the world in 3-D (three dimensions with depth), the brain needs two "cameras". This is covered further in the next chapter. So when we lose the use of one eye, we're just losing one "camera." Our good eye is still sending nerve impulses to the brain as well as it did before.

Your eye doctor will probably have mentioned these parts. This chapter is just a summary, so ask questions! More anatomy is available on the web site, www.asingularview.com. The parts combine to provide vision.

The retina, of course, corresponds to the sensitive film of the movie camera or the CCD of a video camera. And just as the images can be stored on film or disk, so the brain can preserve them in its memory files.

The tiny section of the retina called the fovea (in the middle of the macula) has special properties. It can exercise the finest color discrimination and send the most delicate images with great clarity to the brain. It's the "fine focus" area, and you use all the other eye structures to get this area of the retina in line with the object of interest—muscles, cornea, lens, fovea.

Most of the time people use their cameras for fixed viewing. During the remaining fraction, these "cameras" swivel back and forth, up and down, in a series of incredibly rapid eye move-

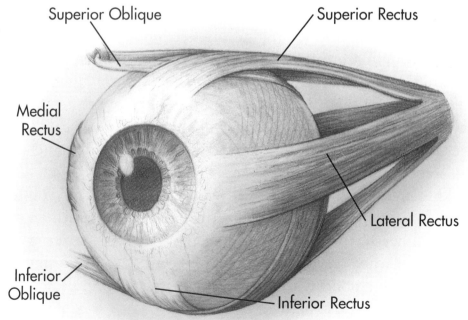

Each eye looks in the direction it is positioned by the six extraocular eye muscles.

ments, scanning various parts of the surrounding scene in two or three "takes" per second. These movements, called saccades, are possible only because the fastest muscles in the body are those muscles directing the eye to where we want to look. These are called the extraocular muscles because they are outside the eyeball and control it.

With two eyes, two slightly different pictures (views separated by the distance between the eyes) are fused together by the brain. The difference in these two pictures is understood by the brain to give a sense of the depth in space—spatial perception in three dimensions—which tells us that things are nearer or farther away.

In short, it is truly a natural optical feat that cannot be reproduced by man's inventions. It's true that a hawk can see better at great distances than a man, and that a cat can see better in the dark. But for all-around viewing purposes, there's certainly nothing better than a human eye.

Except, perhaps, two of them.

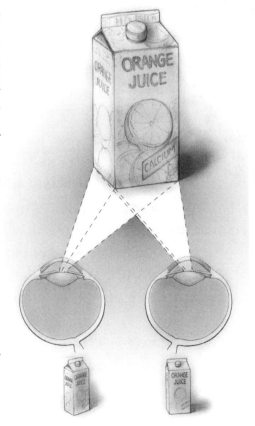

With two eyes, two slightly different pictures are combined in the brain to provide a sense of depth—binocular spatial perception.

Chapter 7

What Has Changed?

WHAT HAPPENS PHYSIOLOGICALLY when you lose one of those two optical marvels with which you've been viewing the world? You know as soon as you step back out into that world that *something* has happened because it seems suddenly to have been transformed into a flat photograph. Your adaptation to this new and uncomfortable environment can be speeded up by an elementary understanding of what's taken place inside of you.

Three things have happened:

1. Your horizontal field of vision has narrowed.
2. Your depth perception has been impaired.
3. Your whole visual system, including brain and motor functions, is in disarray and needs reprogramming so the two can be able to work together.

Other minor effects will be touched on later. But first let's consider these three important ones.

THE VISUAL FIELD

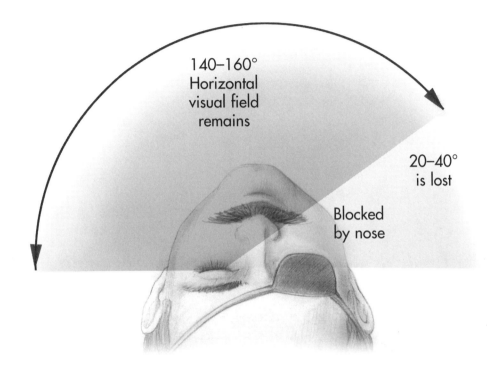

140–160°
Horizontal
visual field
remains

20–40°
is lost

Blocked
by nose

The one-eyed horizontal visual field is not that different—
at most *20% is missing.*

You've literally lost out by a nose here. As we remarked in the last chapter, each eye has a lens capable of taking in everything on the horizon within 180 degrees, or a half-circle.

The horizontal field for one eye will encompass up to 160 degrees, compared with over 180 degrees for normal, two-eyed vision. That bony prominence in the middle of your face called a nose cuts off anywhere from 20 to 40 degrees of that view (depending, naturally, on its size and shape). This was no problem, of course, so long as you had a good eye on the other side of your nose. Each eye was then able to stand guard over that area the other couldn't cover.

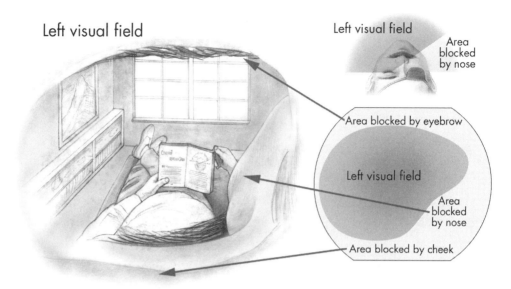

The visual field of the one-eyed person is limited by the eyebrow above, the cheek below, and the nose on the lower edge.

With only one eye, the total field of view once covered by both your eyes has been reduced by 10 to 20 percent, and all of that reduction is on the side of the nonfunctioning eye, your affected side.

The affected side, as you've already surmised from reading about my first difficulties, is where the danger lurks, especially during the early stages of your recovery. Actually, it's more of a nuisance than a danger once you've made adjustments to your new limitation. If the loss of lateral vision seems enormous to you (as it usually does at first), keep in mind that it's really less than many persons with two good eyes see when wearing heavy-rimmed glasses. You'll adjust to it.

Once an Italian Duke of Urbino lost an eye in battle and—being more concerned with fighting than with his appearance—had his surgeon remove the bridge of his nose in order to widen his field of view. This is not recommended as a cosmetic enhancement!

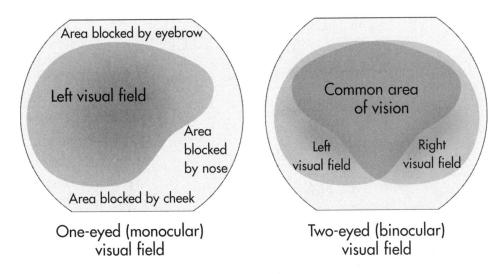

One-eyed (monocular)
visual field

Two-eyed (binocular)
visual field

The view you had with two eyes is really only a little larger.
Mostly what's lost is the binocular vision.

Your *vertical* field of vision (up and down), which totals around 130 degrees, won't be affected. To check this and to keep on the lookout for sneaky glaucoma, your eye doctor may have your field of view checked at regular intervals.

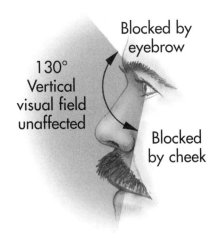

The vertical visual field of the one-eyed is basically unchanged. It is limited by the eyebrow and the cheek.

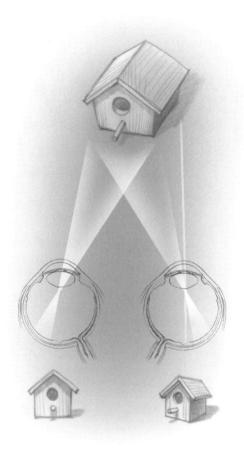

*Retinal disparity—
each eye seeing a
slightly different
image—helps the
brain compute size
and distance
of objects. We one-
eyed people have lost
this mechanism, so we
use other means to
realize three
dimensions.*

DEPTH PERCEPTION

The mechanisms by which we judge the size of an object and its distance from us are much more complex than most people realize.

In part, this is because psychological factors often have an important influence on such judgments. Optical illusions and examples abound.

However, depth perception also involves several pretty sophisticated *physiological* operations. In medical terminology these are known as retinal disparity, convergence and accommodation.

Retinal disparity is the most obvious and widely known of these mechanisms. It depends on an object being viewed with two eyes separated by several inches so that each eye is looking at the same target from a slightly different location at the same moment. One eye sees a little way around to the left. The result: two slightly different images are produced on the two retinas. Before these images are merged into one clear picture, the brain examines the differences and uses them to make a swift computation of the object's size and how far away it is.

Since the differences diminish rapidly with distance, this mechanism is of little use for judging remote objects. The person who no longer has two good eyes doesn't have a chance of using it at all.

Convergence has to do with the merging of these two images produced on the retinas. The effort by the eyes to bring the two images into exact correspondence produces a strain on each eye, and the experienced brain knows how to translate this into a measure of distance. The closer the object, the greater the difference. So the retinal range finder of retinal disparity is coupled with the strain on the converging eye muscles. If you've ever looked cross-eyed at a pencil held in front of your nose, you've experienced this strain at its extreme.

Like the mechanism of retinal disparity, convergence is useful only at relatively small distances (25 feet or less), and only people with binocular vision have it.

Accommodation is a term for the automatic adjustment each eye makes to bring an object into focus. This is accomplished by changing the curvature of the lens, and the muscular effort required doing so is immediately registered on the brain as a measure of distance. Accommodation also includes a change in pupil size and is only useful for nearer objects.

Accommodation is only effective for judging distances up to about six feet; thus it's likely to be the least useful of the three

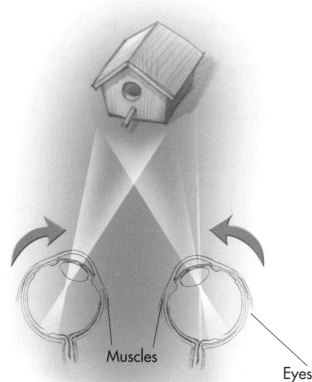

Convergence—the range-finder mechanism—allows the brain to compute distances based on the different angles from which each eye sees an object. The strain on the eye muscles helps make this more accurate.

Muscles

Eyes must turn inward on close objects, strains muscles

mechanisms. When you've lost an eye, however, it's the only one available to you, and so we will cultivate it to its limit. You'll soon learn, however, that there's greater gain in developing new techniques to compensate for the loss of retinal disparity and convergence.

Bear in mind, too, that adaptation is necessary only up to a point. R.L. Gregory of Cambridge University's psychology department notes in his book *Eye and Brain* that all sighted persons "are effectively one-eyed for distances greater than 20 feet." Just like our two-eyed companions using binoculars—after a certain distance, no depth differences can be seen; and

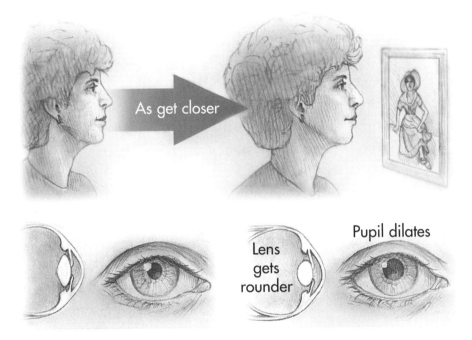

Accommodation—the change in curvature of the lens and pupil size to bring objects into focus—is immediately interpreted by the brain as a measure of distance.

yet some companies sell binocular telescopes for astronomy—there's very little "3-D stereo" to be seen!

There's also a comparison between this and a hearing person losing the use of one ear—the music still comes through fine, but they can no longer tell which direction it's coming from—they have lost the dimensional recognition of 3-D stereo. They have lost "direction," we have lost "distance"—both of which are usually in stereo.

Hmmm, now—I have two nostrils, why can't I tell which direction a smell is coming from? That one is different, because the gases of aromas are dispersed evenly. Maybe a dog can?

THE VISUAL SYSTEM

The relationship between your eyes, your brain and your body is something that has been developing since the day you were born. Seeing is only a part of the visual process that calls for all elements of the system to respond to one another's functions with amazing swiftness and sensitivity.

Even as you read this book, your brain, receiving a signal from your eye, consults its own vast memory bank in order to make a judgment about it. The brain then sends out its commands via the nervous system to activate the body's motor systems. "Turn the page," says your brain, and your fingers obey.

What happens when your brain receives an impaired or different visual message, one for which it has no precedent in its memory bank? To understand how the visual system can be disorganized, let's picture a batter who is about to swing at a pitcher's ball.

He's trained himself to judge the speed and path of the ball by any or all of the three physiological depth-perception processes we've just talked about.

A fourth factor he sometimes brings into his computations is the angle at which the ball is approaching the plate. The angle changes as the ball nears, and the brain has the ability to convert the information on the degree of change into a prediction as to where and when the ball will cross the plate. Having digested all available information, the brain at the proper instant sends out a command to the proper muscles to swing the bat. Then, if all goes well, the ball and bat connect solidly at exactly the right time and place.

But suppose we ask this batter to close one eye and repeat the performance. Only one of the three built-in depth perception techniques—*accommodation*—is now available to him. And as we know, it won't do him any good until the ball is practically on top of him. So he's forced to rely very heavily on information derived from the angle of the ball's approach.

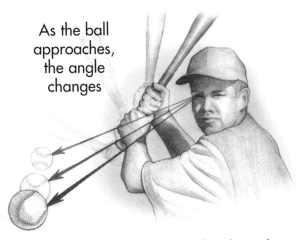

As the ball approaches, the angle changes

A batter unconsciously develops the ability to judge the speed and path of a ball based on the change of angle.

But his techniques for observing the angle have not really been sharpened (as they would be if this had always been the only information available). His brain's file on the subject of that baseball is still small. In short, he'll probably miss the ball until his brain catches up.

Even if he's been a highly skilled ballplayer, a great part of his learned skill will be lost in the transition from dual to single vision. If, instead of just closing one eye experimentally, our batter had actually lost the use of that eye permanently, he'd have to develop a whole new set of skills. He'd have to supply his brain with a whole new complex system of signals and experiences to store up for future reference.

Most amateurs in the same one-eyed situation, however, should certainly be able to get back enough skill to enjoy the game. And many may find, as I often did, that a slight loss of ability can be more than made up for by an increase in effort and attention. In fact, in many less critical sports than baseball, there's no reason why the loss of an eye should be any problem at all.

So far we have considered what happens when a ball player loses one eye. What about the player who is born with only one good eye . . . can he or she excel at the sport?

About two years before the first publication of this book, I heard rumors that Babe Ruth, one of the premier athletes of the twentieth century, played throughout his career with only one good eye. With the help of friends, I was able to find that the information came from New York ophthalmologist, Gerald B. Kara. Dr. Kara examined Ruth a year before his death and has generously shared his findings. His observations are worthy of passing on:

"Babe Ruth was not 'one-eyed' in the true sense of the term. He did have two eyes. However, in the left eye he had amblyopia ex anopsia, which is a congenital condition—he evidently was born with an underdeveloped macula in that eye, which gave him a maximum vision of 20/200. This is insufficient for definitive visual acuity. If that had been his dominant eye, he certainly could not bat or catch a fly ball with it. As it was, Ruth's right eye was dominant, and being a left-handed batter, he saw the pitched ball coming towards him primarily with his right eye. There evidently was just barely enough vision in the left eye to afford him some degree of *stereopsis*. But his fusion was certainly faulty. . . .

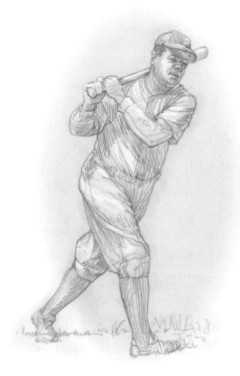

"Ruth spent his early youth

in an orphanage and never really had a sophisticated ophthalmic examination. He told me he was aware of the relatively poor vision in the left eye but 'never did anything about it'. 'Besides,' he said, 'I would never tell those other guys about it!', referring to the other baseball players. He said, 'the problem never bothered me.'"

An Eye on Rembrandt

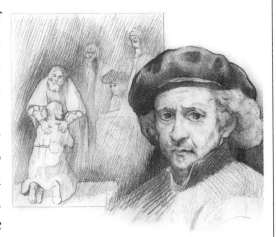

Rembrandt's command of light and darkness makes characters in his paintings appear real enough to touch, from the musketeers setting off on a mission in "Night Watch" to Christ's crumpled figure in "Descent from the Cross", according to an article from the *Boston Globe*.

Margaret S. Livingstone and Bevil R. Conway, neurobiologists at Harvard Medical School, say Rembrandt's many self-portraits reveal that his eyes are focused in slightly different directions, depriving him of the "stero" effect that makes vision three-dimensional. As a result, they argue, Rembrandt would have struggled with depth perception—though he may never have known he had a vision defect.

Some art teachers actually instruct students to close one eye in order to flatten what they see, the researchers write in *New England Journal of Medicine*, explaining their theory about Rembrandt. "Steroblindness might not be a handicap—and might even be an asset—for some artists."

Chapter 8

Getting Back to 3-D

HAVE YOU EVER seen a photographer cover one eye to study a scene before he takes the picture? What he's trying to do, of course, is to view the picture in two dimensions, the way his one-eyed camera will view it.

That's somewhat the way you'd view the world from now on, if you took the loss of one eye sitting still. With your head motionless, you no longer see a little to the right and a little to the left of every object to give it depth. Your eyes no longer strain to bring two slightly different images into correspondence on your retinas. Thus deprived of the two most important physiological means of depth perception—retinal disparity and convergence—what you see is a rather flattened-out scene, much like an ordinary photograph.

Now tilt your head back so that your eye moves up a couple of inches. Something happens. Everything in the room shifts position a little. The edge of the chair in front of you seems to go down a bit, the TV behind it seems to come up a bit, and you now see a bit more of the TV screen. Your brain at once translates the degree of shift into an estimate of the distance between the TV set and the chair, and for an instant you are able to see your surroundings in three dimensions again.

Note that I said "tilt your head"—this phenomenon works whether you are moving your head in any direction. Tilting your head would look to another observer that you are nodding "yes" rather than shaking your head "no"—much more positive!

Perhaps your brain's estimate was off by a hair or a hand: no problem. With practice you're going to become rather accurate at this kind of estimating. In fact, it's going to become a way of life with you.

What has happened? You have created and used the phenomenon of movement in relation to an object, the same technique used by our batter in the last chapter, when he swung at the ball with one eye closed—only the ball was moving, not his eye.

Relative movement in relation to a fixed object is one of the two most important methods by which you're going to win your way back into a three-dimensional world and a normal life. The other method is learning to pick up the subtle clues to depth and distance that artists call *perspective*. Both of these methods are going to be part of your daily living from here on, so let's take a look at each in turn.

RELATIVE MOVEMENT

All of us use this technique constantly to help other methods of depth perception, often without being aware that we're doing it. For the one-eyed person, a grasp of the principles involved is an important shortcut to full adaptation.

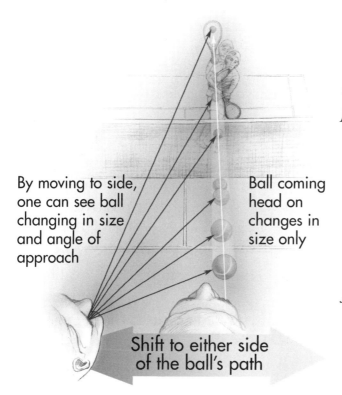

By moving to side, one can see ball changing in size and angle of approach

Ball coming head on changes in size only

Shift to either side of the ball's path

Correct tennis position is suited to the needs of the one-eyed player. It is always to the side, out of the path of the ball. When the ball is coming head on, a quick shift of position provides additional cues to judge where the ball is headed.

One final reference to our batting friend out there on the field: he was able to use the principle of relative movement because he was standing *to one side* of the plate at which the ball was aimed. So the ball sped toward him at an angle, which kept changing as it approached. Without this angle, his brain would have had little information to judge his swing.

Now let's leave the baseball field and move to a tennis court. Here we'll ask you to imagine yourself behind the net with a ball coming directly toward you. As it approaches, there's no change in the angle of its path—just an apparent increase in its size, which is not enough information for your brain to accurately tell where its going.

What do you do to tell where it's going? Shift your position by placing yourself off to the side, just like a coach would tell you. This creates the *angle of approach* your brain needs to compute the ball's motion relative to you. Your chances of whacking the ball with your racket have now improved. You have used a technique; you have met a challenge.

In the absence of binocular vision, relative movement is going to be your prime visual tool in the highly mobile world of driving, walking, boating, skiing, skating and skin diving, and in work involving moving objects or vehicles. Knowing how to create relative movement—when it doesn't occur by itself—is important in getting back to your active life.

One illustration will suffice to show the extreme importance of developing this skill in driving. Every motorist is familiar with the driver who starts to pass you in the left lane, but then slows down and drives neck and neck with you for a long distance. This situation is very irritating to the one-eyed driver. Even though both cars are traveling at highway speed, the relative movement between them is zero. This means that the one-eyed driver has very little in the way of clues to the distance between the two cars.

What's the solution here? Change speed—go a little faster or a little slower than the other car. The result is relative motion and a much-improved ability to judge the distance between the two cars. It's often just that simple to sharpen your depth perception and maneuver yourself out of a dangerous situation.

When viewing a stationary object at short range, one very effective way to produce something akin to relative motion is to move your head quickly to one side. Not only does this create a slight shift of the object against its background (overlapping), it also enables you to have two slightly different views of the same

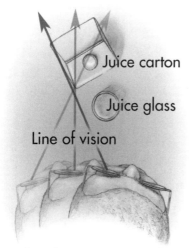

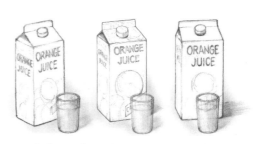

Juice carton

Juice glass

Line of vision

Shifting head position produces
3-D effect by varying perspective
and overlapping of objects

A quick side movement of your head can simulate binocular vision,
especially at close range.

object in such rapid sequence that the brain can interpret them
much the same as it would interpret a double image produced
by two eyes. This is exactly what pigeons and other birds are
doing as they walk with a forward-backward head motion—
they are getting 3-D stereo vision.

I find this rapid head movement one of the handiest tricks
for improving distance judgment up to several feet. And while I
wouldn't advise you to become an obvious swivel-head, I would
suggest that you use your normal head movements as fully as
possible to give your world a third dimension.

PERSPECTIVE

We can turn to the world of art for other important methods of
improving depth perception. Over time, artists have come up
with several ways of showing a three-dimensional world (in space)
upon a two-dimensional canvas or flat sheet of paper. These tricks

can be equally useful to you, if in reverse. That is, in converting your newly flattened-out world (one-eyed, flat pictures) back into round and deep space in your mind (two-eyed, stereo vision of space), these principles can help, with training and practice.

Let's look at some principles. All these techniques can be lumped under the general term "perspective."

Let's stand at a window and ask the great artist Leonardo da Vinci to join us. Leonardo's written descriptions of how he used light, color and shadow to gain realism and depth in his paintings have much to teach us even today. With the old master's help, we notice three important facts about the scene outside our window—our "visual field."

Objects in the foreground take up more of your visual field (or your window space) than objects of the same size in the distance. Cars, which are pretty standard in size, are helpful in this. Leonardo called this "vanishing perspective"—simply said, things that are closer look larger. Even though we know their actual size is the same anywhere, their apparent size is larger when they are nearer to our window.

Colors are another key—they are bolder and brighter nearby; in the distance, they become softer and muted. Also, shadows of nearby objects are sharper and darker. The artist calls this *contrast perspective*. Contrast is lessened as things "fade" into the distance.

Vanishing perspective is another principle noticed as regularly-spaced objects—like telephone poles or fence-posts, for instance—seem to get smaller and closer together, pointing to the horizon. Did you even notice before how straight lines seem to angle together? Like the top ridge of a roof and the sides seem to point together, so even though you know the roof is actually square, the far side looks smaller? "Aha—so *that's* how they do it!" You can use this, too, to estimate distance.

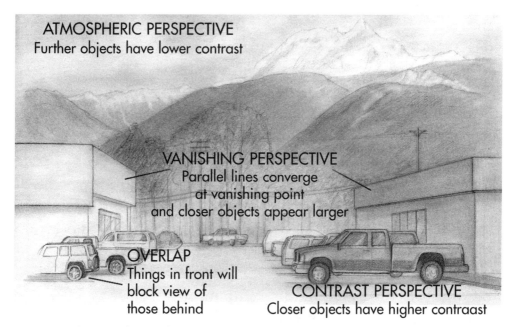

An understanding of artistic principles can help us make sense of the 3-D world around us.

Another color change can be seen in the distance—this can be due to the water vapor in the air as things get bluer in the distance—called *atmospheric perspective* (Leonardo called this *sfumato* or "smoky" perspective). If you really analyze it like an artist does, colors start to drop out pretty quickly in the distance—first yellow, then green, then red (leaving blue, the shorter wavelength of light). The shorter end of the light spectrum scatters more easily, and, sure enough, the mountains become blue, beyond the "purple mountains majesty!" This is related to, though separate from, contrast perspective.

A fourth principle, which is quite simple—so simple that our Leonardo left it out—is that objects *overlap* in space—that is, things that are in front of other objects reduce your view of the ones behind. Simple, right? One car parked down the street blocks the outline of the car parked behind it. When the overlap changes, we know that one of the cars has moved, or we have moved.

These principles are just as useful to the one-eyed person as they are to the artist, because each can be used to improve your depth perception. It's a learning process you can speed up by concentrating on it. As a fringe benefit, you'll find the world more fascinating to view, and you'll know how those artists make their pictures seem "deep enough to walk right into."

While the rules of perspective are simple, using them is sometimes tricky. A car right in front of you takes up much more of your field of vision than another does two blocks away. Since you are familiar with its actual size, you can use its apparent size to estimate its distance from you.

If you know the distance of an object from you—for instance, if you see a round object bobbing in the water at the end of a dock that you know is 50 feet long, it's not hard to estimate the size of that round object as well. However, if you know neither the real distance nor its actual size, you'll have to look for other clues.

A principle used extensively in flying and boating can be extremely useful in these situations. Suppose while you're sailing a boat in a straight line, you see another boat (of unknown size, at an unknown distance) moving on another straight line. You might want to know if its course will eventually cross yours or, worse yet, hit your boat. The best thing to watch is the angle of the other boat in relation to you. If the angle continues to change, the boat will pass clear of you—beware if there's no change in angle. This navigating technique was developed for normal-sighted persons and is even more useful to the person with only one eye. It applies to everyday motion from here out.

Pilots warn their students to "beware of a speck on the windshield that doesn't move, but just keeps getting bigger." That means something is coming straight at you!

Chapter 9

Avoiding Problems and Possible Mistakes

WHEN YOU RETURN to your everyday environment after the loss of an eye, you'll feel like I did, that suddenly problems of all kinds are overwhelming you. Identifying each one is half the battle; developing a technique to cope with each one is the other half.

Nearly all the troubles you're likely to find are traceable to two factors: your loss of depth perception and a reduction in your field of vision. In the previous chapter, we discussed some tricks for regaining depth perception in several situations. But the only way to cope with the cutoff on the sightless side of your nose is to develop the habit of looking around—*before* you move. This means that you will start using your neck more than you used to do!

What follows is a rundown of some specific situations that can bring you bumps, jolts, embarrassments, bruises and even more serious problems if you aren't ready for them—along with a technique for dealing with each of them. Take them one at a time, and return to reread this after a week or so. You'll then be able to have a reminder, and compare that with your new experience.

PUTTING YOUR HANDS TO TASK

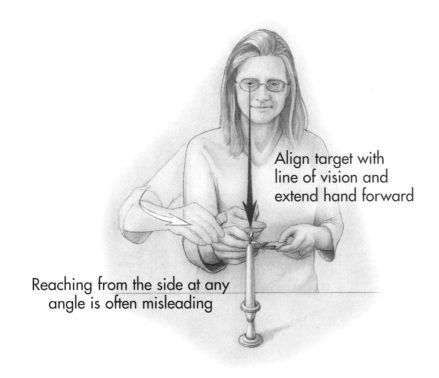

Align target with
line of vision and
extend hand forward

Reaching from the side at any
angle is often misleading

Remember to line up with your target.

The brain knows where all your arms and legs are—this is called *proprioception.* While your brain knows where your hand is, problems may first be apparent in trying to reach things.

One solution that I found useful in the first days was to avoid depending on my brain to figure where my hand was going, and keep my eye on it.

You should have little or no trouble in making contact with an object if you first remember to line up with it and then simply keep on extending your arm and hand until you touch it—it works every time. You will become more attuned to this fact and will soon use this unconsciously. Practice looking at your hand and what's around it—first consciously, then it will become habit, and soon you won't even have to think about it.

This is very simple, can be done without a lot of movement, and no one but you will know you are doing it! Another thing—open your reaching hand and you'll find everything is easier to grasp.

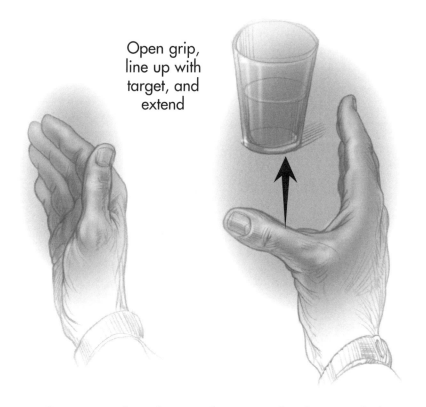

Open grip, line up with target, and extend

Open your hand more than you think is needed.

SHAKING HANDS

Of all my early experiences in adaptation to one-eyed vision, nothing caused me more embarrassment at first than when I reached out to grasp a friendly hand and closed my fingers on thin air— and nothing is more easily avoided with practice.

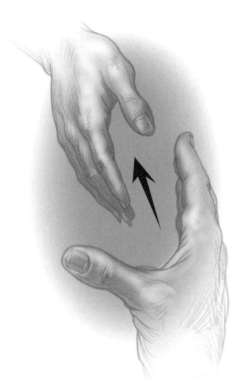

The point to remember is that you don't have to know exactly how far you are from the object you're reaching for in order to connect with it. It's more a question of alignment than judging distance.

To perform this simple act with complete confidence, simply move your hand in a direct line toward your friend's hand, and keep on moving until you connect. They will be moving for yours as well.

The other person's hand will approach yours as well.

POURING

With a little experience, you will gain the distance judgment required to pour water from one container (like a pitcher) into another (like a drinking glass) without missing a drop. Until then, however, it's surprisingly easy to miss completely.

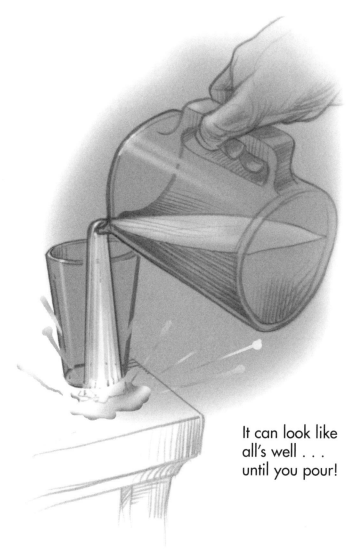

It can look like
all's well . . .
until you pour!

Relying on visual lineup alone may prove inadequate at first.

So in the first few weeks, lightly touch the pitcher to the rim of the glass before pouring. You should also *hold* the glass with your free hand before pouring, as pressure on the edge may tip it, thus spoiling your effort and newfound confidence.

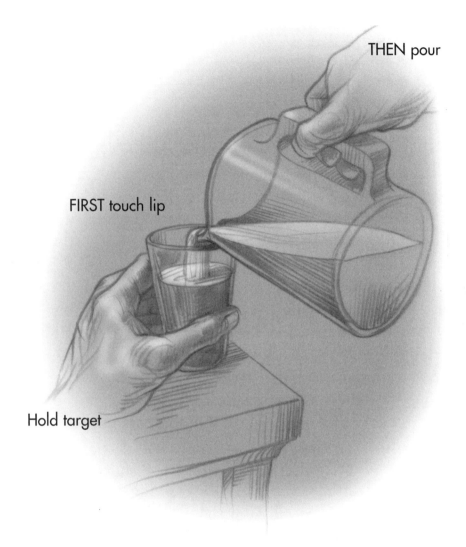

THEN pour

FIRST touch lip

Hold target

Touch your target for now to avoid spills.

As another example of a pouring situation, simply putting sugar in your coffee can seem difficult at first. First we must get the sugar into the spoon, right? Hold the sugar bowl with your free hand, touch the spoon to the rim of the bowl, and dip like you have before. Then (you probably won't have to hold the cup), rest the skinny part of your sugar spoon on the edge of your coffee cup with the sugar over the coffee, turn it over, and all the sugar will get into the cup.

THE COLLISION COURSE

One of the most common complaints of the newly one-eyed is "I'm always bumping into people!" Usually these collisions happen when you make a quick turn toward the affected side—that is, into your new blind spot. Sure, you checked it only a second ago and found that space to be empty, but someone just seemed to appear!

The point is this: "a moment ago" is simply too long a time to account for any and all danger. You need to check that blind spot the very instant you're ready to make your turn. That way no one can take you by surprise. Call it "defensive walking" if you like. It's up to you to make sure that you are safe.

This new habit of checking probably will become natural only after you've had more than a few bumps. If you use it carefully in *all* situations that involve a change of direction, you'll feel more confident and self-assured very soon—particularly where safety is involved, as in swimming, skiing, riding, skating or boating, and most especially in driving. Look both ways, and then back to the first—such as 1) affected side 2) good side 3) affected side.

Before you change lanes on the highway, take a *very* good look around to make sure some small car hasn't crept up and is lurking just outside your field of vision. **Look just before acting** is the point: *knowing* what's going on all around you is your key to safety. There are a few gadgets to help in Chapter 12.

DINING

I've often noticed that a left-handed person will choose a seat at the table where he won't tangle with someone else when they start to eat. For example, if a left-handed person sits to the right of a right-handed person, elbows become weapons, and accidents can be expected. In the same manner, when it doesn't violate a carefully worked-out seating plan, I choose a seat that will favor my good eye. Everyone benefits—the waitperson can approach without fear of a spill, and a hostess won't need to call for a mop.

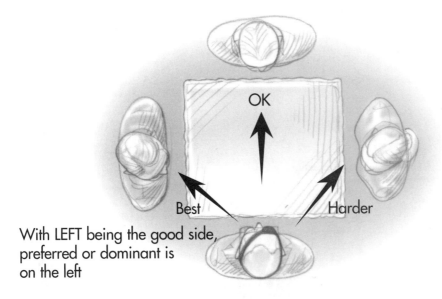

OK

Best   Harder

With LEFT being the good side, preferred or dominant is on the left

Choose your "good" (vision) side first.

My affected side is on the right—I lost my right eye—and I find that if I'm trying to keep up a conversation with someone on my right, the amount of head twisting involved is excessive. This is tiring to me, and may be annoying to them. A fascinating dinner partner may be worth the extra effort. Still, if you can make early arrangements to favor your good side, everyone will be happier.

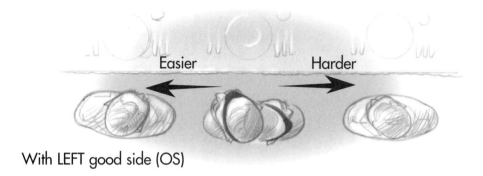

Easier   Harder

With LEFT good side (OS)

It's harder to talk without craning on your affected side.

Remember that the choice of the best seat for your conversation doesn't eliminate other dining dangers. If the meal is being served by a waitperson—especially a skilled, nearly invisible one—they will traditionally approach you from the left, and may be at your affected side the very moment you least expect them. A few bad experiences with spills taught me to take a deliberate look to my affected side before making any unusual or large hand gestures in that direction.

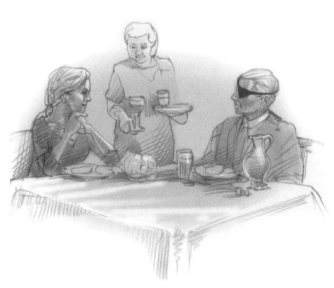

When dining, remember to watch out for waitstaff serving on your affected side and your good side.

STAIRWAYS

Whether you're going up *or* down, *watch that last step*!

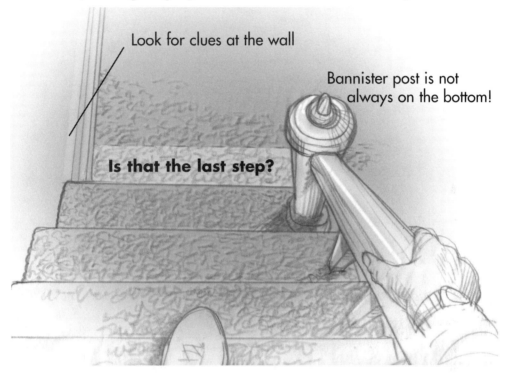

Look for clues at the wall

Bannister post is not always on the bottom!

Is that the last step?

Viewed with one eye, the transition from stairs to floor and vice versa may blend right into one another, especially if they have the same carpeting or finishing treatment and if the light is dim. In either direction, it's all too easy to assume that you've taken the last step and start walking away, only (jolt!) to discover that there was one more . . . and you end up literally on the carpet.

This illusion can be particularly dangerous for the elderly. But anyone who has lost his binocular vision should take that last step gingerly, feeling ahead with his toe and keeping one hand on the handrail.

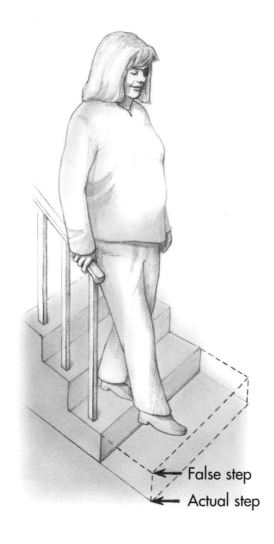

←— False step

←— Actual step

Look out for that last step. It may really be above or below where you think it is, especially when stair and floor coverings are the same.

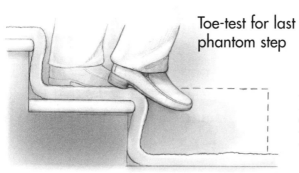

Toe-test for last phantom step

CURBS

A close relative to that last step of the stairway, the curb can be even more treacherous. There is no series of steps to use for estimating the last, and curbs show surprisingly nasty variations in height from one street corner to the next. There are no handrails to hold onto, people are bustling, and a single mistake could easily throw you into the middle of traffic!

After this strong warning, I'm sure you'll immediately start practicing the simple trick I've discovered for estimating the height of a

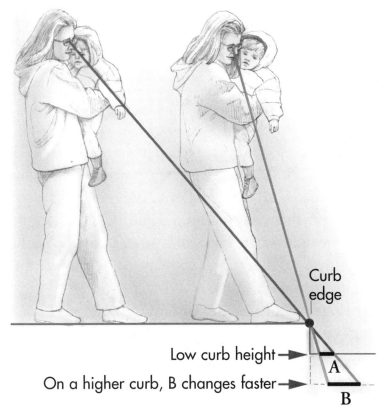

Curb edge

Low curb height →

On a higher curb, B changes faster →

A

B

Use the curb edge as a reference point to judge curb height. For a low curb, segment A will be short compared with B for a higher curb.

curb. It uses the same principle of relative motion that we've already explored: As you approach the street, keep your eye on the edge of the curb so you can observe its relative movement against the background of the street's surface. The higher the curb, the faster this relative motion will appear and the faster it will reveal the street surface. Your brain will have no trouble at all computing these factors, along with your walking speed, and will send you a message telling you just how deep a step to take till you hit the street.

With a little practice (and I suggest that you do your first practicing in a safe place with a handrail as backup) the technique will become so routine that you won't even have to think about it. It'll serve you equally well wherever you have to judge the distance between two horizontal surfaces. Once you've learned it, you can move in the world with assurance, even over rough terrain.

CROSSING STREETS

Now that I've got you to the curb, I'd better alert you to the dangers out there on the street itself. You're well aware, I'm sure, of the dangers traffic poses for a pedestrian with two good eyes. But the special hazard for the one-eyed is the car that comes from an unexpected direction on your affected side. The only way to cope, of course, is to develop the habit of looking both ways at the very last moment, particularly on the affected side with limited peripheral vision.

Beware of intersections where cars are making right *and* left turns. That car that wasn't signaling when you last looked may be turning anyway. Even though you have the right of way, the driver may assume that you'll see him and step aside—especially taxis, let alone buses that assume the right of way by their size alone.

A special danger is the street that you didn't notice was one-way, especially if the traffic is moving *from* your affected side. If you assume you're crossing a normal two-way street and look first to your left, you might easily step off the curb into the path of a car coming on your right.

A vicious form of this danger awaits the one-eyed North American visitor to the United Kingdom where motorists drive on the left. Busy crossings in London have signs on the pavement reminding you to "Look to Right," but elsewhere it's all too easy to step into a deadly situation. Once you've lost your binocular vision, the best advice anyone can give you for making it to the other side of the street is: "Use your head."

THREADING A NEEDLE

When first attempted with one eye, this simple act can seem as difficult as trying to pin the tail on the donkey with both eyes blindfolded. As in most circumstances, patience is key. Don't rage, don't despair. This involves any sort of threading, including shoelaces and, again, it's a matter of alignment. Here's a technique that works:

1. Cut the thread at an angle with a very sharp pair of scissors or a razor blade to make sure there's no fuzz on the end. Sharpen that point by moistening it and drawing it between your fingers.
2. Hold the needle toward the light and steady your hands together by touching one on the other.
3. Wipe the point of the thread back and forth across the needle, slowly withdrawing it until it just barely misses the needle. The trick is to get the tip as close as possible to the eye before the final step.
4. Now center the point of the thread on the eye of the needle and push it through.

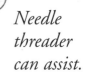

Needle threader can assist.

You can find a simple needle-threading device in any sewing/fabric store that will make the job easier—especially if you also apply the techniques listed above.

CRAFTS AND ART

Hand steadying (resting one on the other) is useful here, though the main way to put anything where you want it is to line it up with your eye and extend your hand (until the brush hits the canvas, needle hits the cloth, glue hits the glass, etc.). This will become second nature soon, and, in repetition, the distance to the surface will become known to your brain.

TARGET SHOOTING

Target shooting with a rifle, or hunting with a shotgun, are sports that normally call for the use of only one eye. Yet this poses a challenge for those in our circumstances. For instance, the right-handed shooter usually holds the stock against the right shoulder, places the left foot forward, and sights with the right eye. If the affected side is on the right, this may seem impossible—to lean over and sight with the left eye, when the stock seems to prevent it. However, like all tools, this can be customized. While some may find this unnecessary and merely lean over, angling the good eye upwards to the sighting plane, this angling may require a lowering adjustment in the comb of the stock.

For using a standard long gun, perhaps it would be best to simply shoulder it on the good side—this is called "switching" and works well. One precaution: automatic ejectors generally throw hot brass to the right of the shooter. If you are switching, this could throw it *toward* you, possibly causing injury, so choose your shoulder arms carefully.

The first time you try this, everything will feel all wrong. Your scores will show a dramatic drop, particularly if you're shooting at a live or moving target. "It'll never work," you'll quickly conclude. Yet many people have brought their scores back up to their old levels with persistence.

One enthusiastic advocate of switching is my friend Jack Fletcher, a photographic specialist with the National Geographic Society. An avid skeet fan, Jack had been shooting for years without ever having achieved a perfect score. Then he lost his dominant right eye and had to find an instructor to teach him how to shoot off his left shoulder. The training was so successful that Jack has since shot not one but several perfect scores.

EXERCISE WITH A BALL

Practically all the skills called for in the simple acts of everyday

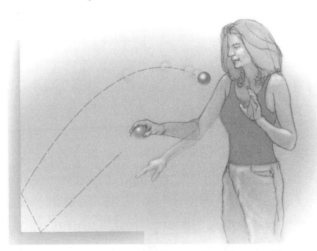

living with one eye can be sharpened by exercising with a ball. Simply bouncing a ball off a wall for a few minutes each day or playing catch with a friend can improve your visual skills enormously. So can any of the ball games like tennis, baseball, or basketball.

All these activities demand accommodation and call for judgment of angle, size, distance, relative motion and timing. And all the gains you make in these activities can be carried over into your daily routines.

Chapter 10

In the Driver's Seat

UNDER NORMAL CIRCUMSTANCES, there's no reason why you can't learn or continue to drive with only one eye. There *are* a few situations in driving that you may find a bit bothersome and that will require some special attention.

I'm sure you'll have no more trouble than I did on the open highway. Actually, most of your visual problems will be on narrow, crowded streets, and at times when you're driving slowly and trying to judge distances on either side of you. One difficult feat, until you're accustomed to monocular vision, is threading your way through a narrow street between parked cars without scraping any paint off them. Three ways to handle this (in increasing order of difficulty) are:

1. Follow the car ahead of you. With this tester to tell you if it's safe to go on, you'll have no problem (unless you're driving a half-ton truck and following a subcompact car or vice versa).

2. If there's no car ahead of you, ask your passenger to assess the right while you concentrate on the left.

3. If you have no passenger, look ahead to make sure you have adequate clearance, and concentrate all your attention on driving close to the line of cars on your driver's side—with your head out the window if necessary—thus the right will take care of itself.

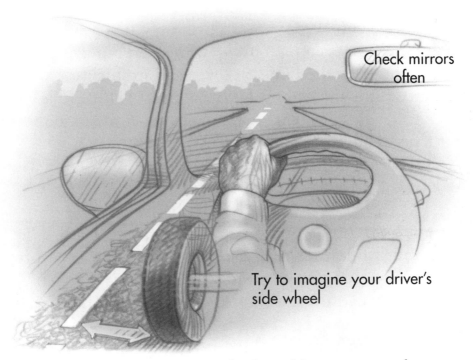

Check mirrors often

Try to imagine your driver's side wheel

Try to imagine your wheels and bumpers—and keep to the driver's side.

A more nerve-racking variant of this is the narrow two-way street where you have to make room for an oncoming car without touching the cars parked to your right. Your alternatives in this problem are:

1. Drive close to the center line, so as to leave plenty of room between yourself and the parked cars. If there is no center line, project an imaginary line onto the street and try to use it the same way.
2. If this proves too difficult, stop your car at the widest available space and simply wait for him to pass.

Auto safety engineers could make a real contribution by requiring that corner posts on all new cars be designed to minimize visual obstruction. The wide posts popular on some cars today can block out an astonishingly large swath of the scene to the rear, even for a driver with good binocular vision. When sight is limited to one eye, the problem is severely aggravated, and the only solution I know is a flexible neck. Frequent head movements will enable you to see around the obstruction and avoid any danger.

PARKING

One of the things you sooner or later must learn is to accept your limitations and exercise patience with yourself. If you know what you can't do, you may save yourself a lot of pain and frustration by trying to avoid certain situations altogether.

Before my accident I prided myself on my parking ability, so it took some frustrating experimentation to convince me that I'm just not as adept anymore.

I find that maneuvering my car into a tight space in a parking lot between two other cars—and knowing that the slightest bump can result in costly damage thanks to incredibly bad car design—is often more aggravation than it's worth.

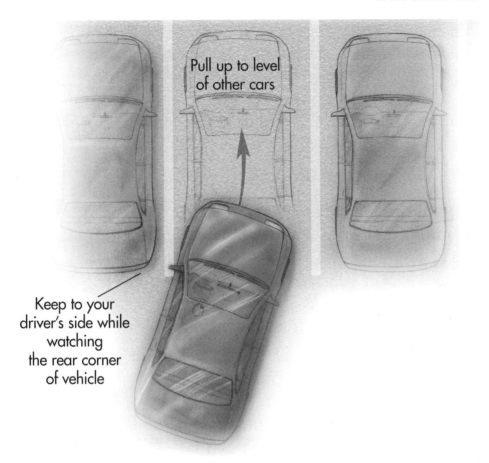

Pull up to level
of other cars

Keep to your
driver's side while
watching
the rear corner
of vehicle

*Keep to the driver's side in all tight spaces, and the
other side will take care of itself.*

If there's a passenger with me, I have no hesitancy about putting them to work to help me clear the other cars. When I'm
alone, I sometimes get out of my car to survey the situation and
plan my maneuvers with precision. But more often, if there's
time, I'll try to find a wider slot or even go considerably out of
my way to find a spot that I can get into and out of with ease.
Patience prevails.

Maybe parking will be a snap for you. I often marvel at the
aplomb of a garage attendant in my office building. While wear-

ing a patch over one eye, this young man races the cars through underground mazes, jockeying this one and that one from rear to front, all with the greatest assurance and enjoyment. Whether his monocular vision has anything to do with the dents and scratches customers claim they sometimes find on their cars, I'm not in a position to say. But I wish I knew the secret of his assurance.

Some trucks place a vertical rod to indicate to the driver where the bumpers are when they cannot be seen. This may be an option though its another aerial to remove at the car wash. You'll soon have an idea of where your bumpers are, and the car once again will feel like an extension of your body. Just give everything a wide berth for now.

I have developed a trick or two that you can use for snuggling into your own garage without hitting the rear wall. Turn on the headlights, even in daytime, and watch the pattern the beam makes on the wall as you approach it: A curved line of light moves downward as you approach the wall. By putting a marker—a piece of tape for example—on the wall when the car is safely resting with its light on in the garage, you can stop the car just as the line of light reaches the marker. I use this little trick on a daily basis and find that it is very precise. I can stop the car so the front bumper is within an inch of the desired distance from the wall.

A friend uses another simple device that gives equally good results. She suspends a tennis ball from the garage ceiling and adjusts the length of string until the ball just touches the sloping windshield when the car reaches the desired distance from the wall ahead. This would aid anyone, regardless of the condition of their vision.

An alternative and effective aid is a short strip of tape

placed vertically on the side wall of the garage nearest to your good eye to mark your stopping point.

PICKING A CAR

When you're in the market for a new car, you'll want to consider several features that are more important to you than to the average car buyer. These include field of vision, size, convenience and all-weather capability.

For visibility, check whether the car's design allows you to see all around. Do corner posts obstruct your view and does curved glass distort what you see? Do you sit high enough to see over the hood and trunk? Does the inside rearview mirror give you a wide-angle view?

Good lights for night driving are important, and, fortunately, today's cars come equipped with excellent lighting systems. I suggest you have halogen lamps installed. You can optimize performance of lights by making sure they are kept clean and properly aligned. I'd suggest adding fog lamps, depending on your area.

Your car's size makes a big difference when it comes to driving ease. Although there is some trade-off in comfort and possibly safety, you should test drive a smaller car and see how much extra room you have for parking or maneuvering through tight traffic. You may find driving a peppy little car a lot more fun, even if it seems your groceries fill up the back seat. "Land yachts" are harder to negotiate.

You will find it worthwhile to have a washer, wiper and defogger for the rear window as well as the windshield. They can add a lot to your peace of mind. Mine get a lot of use. Make sure you regularly replace your windshield wiper blades, or get some that are oversize.

Other innovations will come along, including video cameras to aid in backing up and satellite locator systems.

There is no reason why you can't safely drive a minimally equipped car, but driving one with the features I've described can increase your comfort and enjoyment. And with a car like this in bad weather, you'll be able to see more with your one eye than most of the drivers on the road.

DRIVEN TO DISTRACTION

With the advent of cellular phones and other distractions, driving is dangerous enough for the binocular. You and I need to pay particular attention to decreasing distractions while driving. Otherwise, we cannot do the head movements we need to.

- Consider getting remote audio controls for your car stereo—some models now have these on the steering wheel, which you can adjust by feel.
- Get a built-in phone or a hands-off system from your phone company. (Some states actually require this.)
- Install a rearview mirror with a wider angle.
- Give yourself a few minutes for your vision to adapt when you are about to drive at night.
- Avoid heavily tinted glass.
- Never eat or drink hot liquids while the car is moving.
- Keep your head moving.
- Check your mirrors often.
- Visually check to see that your turn signal is working— you cannot always hear the sound.

- Watch for flashing lights of emergency vehicles—you cannot always hear the sirens.
- Keep looking to the road and your surroundings.
- Clean all glass regularly, inside and out, including lights.
- Watch those all-important blind spots—especially behind and to the right (in North America), but anywhere on your affected side.
- Adjust mirrors to cover as much of your periphery as possible. You do not have to see the side of your car in the side mirrors—focus just off your panels. Obtain and adhere additional small convex mirrors on your side mirrors if coverage is patchy.
- Your horn is your one way to communicate with drivers around you—use it! But it only takes a short beep.
- Pledge to yourself to travel through animals on the road or ignore them completely. A swerve can put you out of control, putting you and your passengers at risk.
- Keep a steady grip on the wheel, but relax your elbows—your driving will be smoother, and you will arrive less tense.
- Cruise control will ease tension on a long trip.
- Choose a route that offers less traffic congestion.
- Check both ways and then again to the first direction (for instance, right, then left, then right).
- Be confident by being aware of everyone around you—surprises are not fun.
- Keep spare glasses (with reflection-free coating) in the car so they are always with you.
- Above all, practice patience—driving is frustrating enough. Let that other car zoom around. They'll be the ones getting ticketed!

Chapter 11

The Active Life

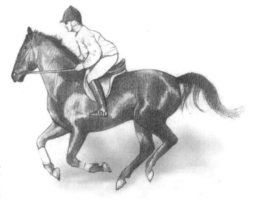

ANYONE WHO FEELS that the loss of an eye marks the end of taking part in sports activities should consider the case of Sue Moran, radio and TV personality, fashion model, committee-woman, and mother of six. Mrs. Moran's 10-year bout with a corneal inflammation ended with the loss of her right eye.

"It hasn't changed my life," she says. "I'm still doing all the things I enjoy and still coping with the endless demands that come with a large family and a country home."

Among the things Mrs. Moran enjoys is riding in competitions such as the International Horse Show in Washington. She also enjoys fox hunting, swimming, skiing and bird watching—all sports that make heavy demands on visual perception and judgment.

Because the speeds involved demand lightning judgments, skiing would seem to require the ultimate in visual perception. Yet ski-jumper Jerry Martin from Minnesota has proved that top-level, competitive skiing is really possible with one eye.

Martin lost the sight in his right eye when a nail he was pounding into brick bounced back and struck his cornea. Although he expects to eventually regain normal sight with a transplant and a contact lens, he has done some amazing things in the meantime. Six weeks after his injury, he was jumping again. And he was doing it so well that within year he won the tryouts for the U.S. Olympic team. (He failed to win a medal at the Olympics, but he did place higher than any other American.)

Commenting on his winning tryout performance, Martin said: "My doctor told me depth perception would be the biggest problem. In ski jumping, you need it for taking off and for landing, but you're only affected at a distance of about 10 feet. I've been jumping a long time and I land more by feel than by sight, so I wasn't worried about that. I wanted to prove to myself that I could keep jumping with one eye. That actually gave me a little extra push."

In contrast, Sandy Duncan, the TV comedy star who lost the sight in one eye, gave a magazine reporter a hilarious account of her efforts to learn to ski. Time after time while standing and talking with her instructor, she'd suddenly find herself starting to slide down the slope: "Finally, we figured it out. Because of this eye thing I can't determine the direction the slope falls. I would think I was standing across the fall line when in fact I was headed straight down the slope." But with the same determination she's shown in coping with her handicap, Ms. Duncan added, "I'll learn."

Kirby Puckett, Hall of Famer formerly with the Minnesota Twins baseball club, and Dick Vitale, the sports announcer, are among sports figures who are monocular, as is Sugar Ray

Leonard—world champion boxer in multiple weights—who sees out of only one eye and retired when a retinal detachment threatened his good eye.

As you test yourself out in the sports that have always given you pleasure, there are a few important physical and psychological factors to keep in mind. From a purely physical standpoint, those sports in which the motion takes place in two dimensions rather than three—bowling, billiards, croquet, skee-ball, and shuffleboard, for example—would be the easiest to remaster. Since the object of play is confined to a single flat plane, the simple visual judgments demanded in these sports can be handled with one eye just about as well as with two.

In three-dimensional sports, monocular vision presents more of a challenge, and your difficulties will be determined by a whole complex of factors. A basketball, for instance, will be easier to manage than a handball; you'll miss less often with a racket than with a bat; a fast game like field hockey or volleyball will come a lot harder than a slower one like badminton.

Racquetball is a fast game, as is squash, but you'll be able to play them. Before you do, though, let me give you a special word of warning. This popular wall-court sport accounts for a number of eye injuries far out of proportion to the number of its participants. I don't condemn the sport and say it should be avoided, but whoever plays it should know the risks involved and take suitable precautions with protective eyewear made with polycarbonate lenses. In most clubs this eyewear is now required before play. The risk of injury is so great that Canada passed a law that requires racquetball players to wear eye guards.

Players with normal vision ought to wear nonprescription protective eyewear specifically made for sports. A player with only one eye shouldn't venture onto a court without the best eye protection available. Regular prescription glasses with impact-resistant lenses can help somewhat in case of an accident, but aren't nearly as effective. Actually, injuries have more often involved the glasses' frames than broken lenses. And with one eye now, the best is never too good for you.

But given the right psychological mindset, no sport is beyond the capabilities of the person who has lost an eye, nor is there any reason to give up those that have always brought you enjoyment. The main thing to remember is that some sports call for a longer period of relearning than others, and during this period you're competing only with yourself.

RUNNING, HIKING, CLIMBING, CYCLING

For competing with yourself, running is still a great all-round workout, but you may find that using machines in a health club is challenging. Take your time. Even two-eyed runners find it tough to get on and off the treadmill. Keep that head moving! Running outside is simply a matter of using the tips for walking/hiking—but at a faster pace—so traffic awareness becomes essential.

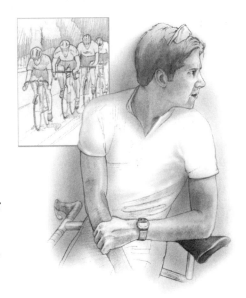

The main potential problem in hiking is judging if "that branch" is going to hit your face. Using protective glasses and caution removes the danger. Use of a hiking staff helps anyone, especially in balancing over river rocks. Walk on top of the rocks, not between. Using a sighting compass and map is no problem, since it's a one-eye function, but using an axe in camp may prove daunting. Extend the axe to touch the wood first, then try to repeat that in your swing. Same thing in golf.

There's no problem in climbing—just start finding grips by putting your hand out and extending—just like meeting a handshake. Some practice in a climbing gym helps.

This psychological stance may be a little harder to acquire in such games as tennis and baseball, in which competition can be a primary goal. If you find any of these too frustrating, why not try making your comeback, initially, in sports that have well-established handicaps, like golf. Those that pit you against your own record, like running, biking, archery or rifle practice. Therefore, you can engage in sports purely for fun and exercise—as well as for competition when you want it—such as water sports.

SWIMMING

This most popular of all water sports is virtually unaffected by the limitations of monocular vision. And this is true not only of surface swimming, but also of underwater swimming with snorkel or scuba gear.

Underwater distance judgments are difficult even with normal eyesight because water bends the light differently from the way air does. Moreover, most underwater masks limit the field of vision so much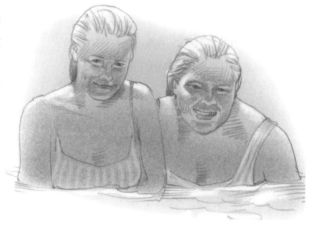

that it makes no difference whether you have one eye or two. So if this activity appeals to you, it's one of the best ways to get back in the swim.

One thing to mention here is that Prevent Blindness of America reports that swimming and watersports account for the second-highest incidence of eye injury. However, the fact that so many participate in one way or another modifies the impact of this statistic.

DIVING

You'll encounter no special problems here either, unless you wear an artificial eye. The sudden pressure when you strike the water, particularly in a high dive, can dislodge the prosthesis. A pair of underwater goggles is the answer. To safeguard your good eye, make sure the lenses are high-impact and shatter-resistant.

FISHING

Although some distance judgments are involved in casting a lure, the distances are beyond the range where binocular vision is any real help. Out on the Bahama flats, I've watched my one-eyed friend Clarke Daniel, with all the skill and precision of a native bonefish guide, drop his shrimp-baited hooks time after time directly in front of the quarry.

The chief danger is having a wild cast put a hook into your eye. This happens mostly as a self-inflicted injury, but a companion can be just as dangerous. Lewis Williams Douglas lost an eye this way while serving as U.S. ambassador to Britain. With only one good eye, you simply can't afford to take that chance, so always wear protective glasses—even if you don't need glasses to correct your vision—with high-impact, shatter-resistant lenses.

WATER SKIING AND SURFING

These sports, though difficult in themselves, pose absolutely no special problems for the one-eyed individual. Impact with the water can displace a prosthesis, though, so goggles are still a good idea.

SAILING, MOTORBOATING

Just a few points for the newly monocular to remember. The danger in jumping from dock to boat and vice versa can be lessened by following the sailor's advice: "One hand for the boat."

A useful device for all skippers, but particularly the one-eyed, is the "telltale"—bits of yarn placed on the shrouds or at the luff to indicate the relative direction of the wind and help obtain the proper trim.

CANOEING, KAYAKING, ROWING

Since you are almost always in motion in these activities, relative motion is easy to use, as your view is almost always informed by a spatial sense. 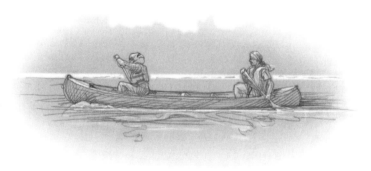 Problems may arise mostly in getting in and out, but these are common to all participants. When landing the boat, keep your head moving.

Chapter 12

Let Technology Help: Gimmicks and Gadgets

HOW DO YOU turn a handicap into an asset?

One way is by taking full advantage of all the marvelous gadgetry created to compensate—even overcompensate—for every imaginable deficiency. Many persons deprived of binocular vision have found that one eye plus a gadget plus a little practice result in a better performance than had been thought possible with two eyes unaided. So let's examine some of the aids and instruments you may find helpful. Almost all of these are also useful for your two-eyed friends.

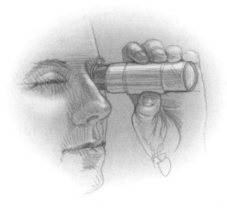

Almost all gadgets will help your two-eyed friends as well.

EYEGLASSES

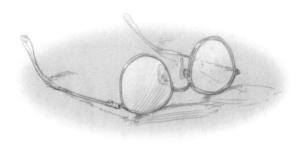

When you've lost one eye, it becomes imperative to protect the surviving one and to enhance its vision to the greatest practicable degree. Of course, only an eye specialist can tell you whether you need glasses and prescribe the corrective lens for you. But there are some considerations to keep in mind when you go to get the prescription filled. There have been quite a few developments in eyeglasses since Ben Franklin invented bifocals in the 18th century.

One of the greatest improvements is the safety standard set by the U.S. Food and Drug Administration. All eyeglasses, including nonprescription sunglasses, must be impact-resistant. This means that the lenses must be able to withstand the impact of a steel ball, the size of a marble, dropped from a height of 50 inches.

To meet this requirement, eyeglass manufacturers began using special plastic or heat-hardened crown glass for their lenses. These materials made glasses more expensive, but the amount is small compared to the added protection they give your eyes, especially if you've already used up your "spare."

The most dramatic improvement in lens material came with the development of a polycarbonate material that far exceeds the impact strength required by law. I wrote to one vendor for information and they sent me a sample lens made of the polycarbonate material. While the specifications were impressive, I wanted first-hand evidence that the material could withstand a severe blow. My experiment was very unscientific: I took the lens to my workshop, put it on the bench, and covered it with a thin cloth to catch any fragments. I gave it a good whack with my three-pound, short-handled sledge hammer. The hammer bounced off. Next I gave the hammer all I had. This time the heavy hammer bounced nearly a foot, and on examining the lens, I found no evidence of fragments or scratching. It's hard to conceive of an accident situation that would cause this material to fracture.

Your visual field, as you know, has already been reduced, and for some activities you certainly won't want to cut it down any more. So choose eyeglass styles accordingly. Glasses with heavy frames, for instance, may be fine for reading, but they cut off so much of your field that they constitute a severe and totally unnecessary handicap when you're driving a car, watching a ball game, or engaging in any other activity that calls for a panoramic view.

Thin-rimmed or rimless glasses cut this problem to a minimum, and a contact lens eliminates it altogether. The crescent-shaped half glasses that many people use for reading are also good in this respect, since you get an unobstructed view over the top of the lens.

Wire-frame glasses do not reduce your visual field excessively, but they're dangerous if you wear them while playing sports. If the glasses receive a hard blow, the sharp wire can severely damage an eye. There have been reports of this kind of accident. At least one manufacturer offers a safe and sturdy alternative: A tough nylon thread in a groove at the circumference of the lens holds the lens in

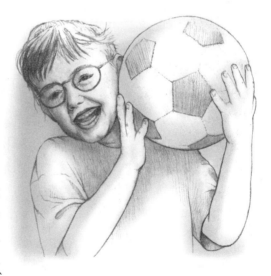

Plastic-frame glasses are recommended for sports activities

place. At no point does the glass touch metal. The result is a strong construction with minimum obstruction to peripheral vision.

The relatively new titanium frames are extremely flexible and seem light and comfortable, but they offer little protection, if simply due to these qualities.

There are special frames for sports use, featuring a headband that keeps them from being knocked off—a type any sailor who has lost a pair of glasses overboard appreciates greatly.

A wide variety of eyewear is now available for those who need protection in active sports such as hockey, football and squash.

Prevent Blindness of America lists basketball as having the highest incidence of sports-related eye injuries. Kareem Abdul-Jabbar popularized the look of protective glasses long ago, so don't hesitate to wear them.

By the way, there are some professional basketball players who are monocular as well, notably Eddie Shannon of the University of Florida, who now plays in Europe and is a standout.

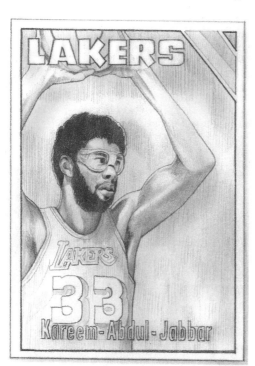

These glasses have a tough plastic wraparound frame with an adjustable headband and can be fitted with prescription lenses of your choice. Sometimes called "combat glasses," their use is not limited to sports, and they can well be used on jobs that present hazards to the eyes. A particular advantage to the monocular is the wraparound design of some models, which offers an exceptionally wide angle of view.

You can also choose from a variety of lens tints and coatings designed for special purposes. For example, a yellow tint absorbs blue light and can be useful when maximum haze penetration or sharpened contrast is needed.

Some lenses are treated to darken when sunlight hits them, so the wearer needn't change glasses when going out in the sun or coming back indoors. But if used under certain conditions, these "photochromic" lenses may pose a problem. Be aware that the windshield inside a car or in an aircraft cockpit may not allow the lenses' sensitive material to be activated, and the wearer isn't getting the protection needed.

A more serious problem is the time it takes photochromic lenses to clear when light conditions change from bright to dim. Some of the lenses never become more than 80 percent clear, which make them unsuitable for night driving. You can imagine the shock you'd get when driving from sunlight into a tunnel. Even in the daylight-to-dusk period the lenses may not change fast enough and, unfortunately, this kind of change is too gradual to warn the wearer that vision is being impaired. Future photochromic lenses may avoid these pitfalls.

There is a nonreflective lens coating that not only makes the wearer's eyes more visible to others but reduces distracting reflections and ghost images. Because most of the light passes through the lens instead of being reflected away, the wearer gets a clearer view. I have found coated lenses very helpful for night driving.

Attempts have been made to extend peripheral vision on the side of the missing eye by optical means. So far as I have been able to determine, a practical and affordable solution to this problem has not yet reached the market. The tiny rearview mirrors that bicycle riders clip on to their glasses extend vision, but on the wrong side. Prism glasses that are offered as a solution may actually be a danger to your good eye in an accident.

I mention these developments in eyewear not to recommend some and tell you to avoid others, but to make you aware of them and better able to discuss your needs with a professional. And remember that whatever type of glasses you're buying—to safeguard your single precious eye, be sure it has nonshatterable lenses that meet or exceed the legal requirements.

Just a word that may save you some money when you buy glasses: Many retail suppliers of eyewear allow for the fact that a monocular customer needs only a single prescription lens, and they adjust their charges accordingly. Others charge full price. Next time you have a lens prescription filled, don't hesitate to ask for a price adjustment. There may not be many advantages to being one-eyed, but this is one of them. Don't expect 50 percent off your eye exam!

EMERGENCY "GLASSES"

Ever get caught in front of a telephone book on the road with no glasses to keep the print from blurring? Here's an emergency measure I picked up and have often been thankful for.

Take a small piece of cardboard or paper—a business card is big enough—and punch a tiny hole in it with a pin or a bent paper clip. Now place your eye against the hole, hold the small print about six inches from your eye, and read. What you've got is a lens that operates on the same principle as a pinhole camera. You may not want to read a long book this way, but it works in an emergency.

MAGNIFIERS

The loss of an eye can become much more of a problem if

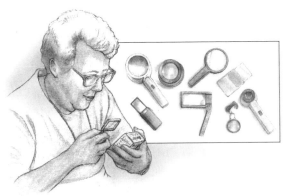

Several types of magnifiers can make reading tasks easier.

vision deteriorates in the surviving eye. A normal kind of deterioration affecting many adults is a decreasing ability to focus on near objects. This is called *presbyopia.* According to Dr. Michael Berenhaus, presbyopia can reach a point where the ability to read small print or to perform very close work is challenging even with corrective lenses.

A magnifying glass can often solve the problem simply, and there's a wide selection available, ranging from small pocket versions to large desk units. Industrial models are mounted on stands so both hands are free to work beneath the glass.

Many units combine a magnifier and a light source, such as a flashlight behind the lens or a fluorescent tube encircling it. There are models for yachtsmen, jewelers, artists, seamstresses, teachers and just ordinary people who want to be able to read a number in the telephone book. The Fresnel lens magnifying sheet, which lies flat on a reading surface, is very inexpensive and can fit in your purse or wallet. Lighted versions are often found in bookstores.

CAMERAS

Today's cameras are no problem for a monocular person. If your camera is manual, you will be able to focus it as well as ever. Most cameras are now automatic or digital, so you will find this unchanged. Photography is hard enough to master, so check out the owner's manual to perfect your photos. Cameras, including digital and video cameras are all monocular anyway, so you may actually be better at using these than your binocular friends!

RANGEFINDERS, MIRRORS AND OTHER OPTICAL AIDS

Being deprived of binocular depth perception gives the one-eyed person a special interest in estimating distances using whatever aids available. This seems desperately essential at first, while you are healing. And your loved ones may spend a lot of money, thinking these actually are what you need. However, you need them *only* if you want or like the technology, and you will soon find that these are really unnecessary, given, as described earlier, that even binocular depth perception is rather inaccurate after about 20 feet.

Everyone can gain by looking through a telescope at nature or using a rangefinder to calculate a golf distance, but you will need these no more than anyone else. Even though binoculars are unnecessary, they are widely available and relatively inexpensive. A good compact telescope is good for anybody, though the folded prism type can be more awkward to handle than the slightly longer version. If you are looking for one of these, do yourself the favor of getting a good brand with relatively high magnification and a soft eye cup—it's worth the cost difference to get quality optics. Your appreciation of the world around you will be enhanced, as it will for your loved ones.

In golf as well as other activities requiring distance judgments, the one-eyed player is only at a disadvantage when short distances are involved. And most of this game is solved using alignment techniques already mentioned. The rangefinders touted by the technology fanatics and well-meaning family member might be just as useful to persons with normal binocular vision, since they cannot tell the distances well either. You may find, as I did, that these only draw attention to your condition.

Many gadgets are available for raising your eyepower. These are useful to everyone, regardless of binocularity, and you will need them no more than anyone else. If you search the Internet, you'll find a wide variety of instruments made to be used with one's eye—telescopes, microscopes, loupes and monoculars, to name a few examples. If you are going to get only one of these gadgets,

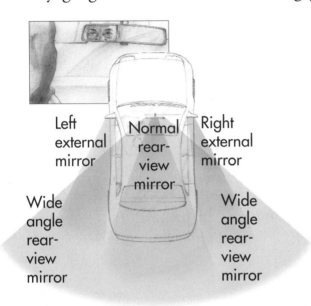

Left external mirror — Normal rearview mirror — Right external mirror — Wide angle rearview mirror — Wide angle rearview mirror

A wide-angle rearview mirror can really help—as a matter of fact, all sorts of mirrors help.

look into a laser tape measure. It is accurate to several wavelengths of light for distances as close as 12 inches up to 40 feet. Now that may be worth looking into!

LARGE PRINT

You've probably noticed that this book is printed in larger than usual type (as I mentioned in the first pages). Although a normal single eye will typically have no more of a problem coping with even fine print than a pair of good eyes, the larger print is used here because some readers may be recovering from a recent eye loss or other associated vision problems as they heal. Two-eyed individuals have the benefit of binocular summation, where the brain adds these images from each eye. For those with a continuing low-vision problem, there is a whole world of books, newspapers, magazines and other publications printed in a type size somewhat larger than you see here.

There has been a virtual explosion of material published in large print. For best sellers and many new books coming on the market, printing of regular and large print editions is now done at the same time, no longer delayed by a year, as when this book was first written. Most public libraries now have extensive collections of large-print books and have information on how to obtain books they don't stock, all available free of charge through Interlibrary Loan programs.

MEASURING TOOLS

It's the little distances that are tough, remember? The inches, feet and yards. So I keep an extra supply of ordinary measuring tools near at hand—tape measures, yardsticks, rulers, etc. Being forced to make exact measurements instead of guessing will bring the blessings of precision into many jobs you perhaps once didn't do nearly so neatly and nicely.

Go ahead and look into the laser measuring tool mentioned earlier. You will agree with builders that it is invaluable.

LIGHTING

I strongly believe that special kinds of lighting can do much to aid

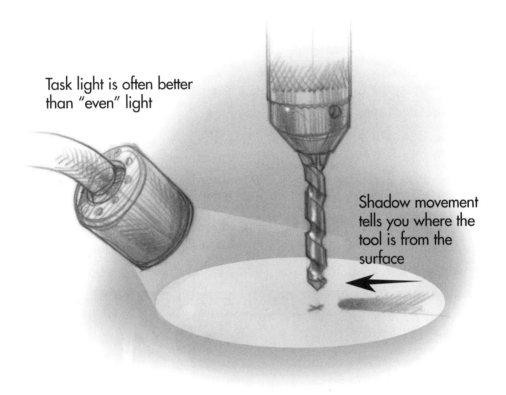

Task light is often better than "even" light

Shadow movement tells you where the tool is from the surface

Look at the shadows to tell you distances in close-up work.

anyone's vision. Our uses of the light are just a bit different from most people's.

Since I do a lot of close work myself, I've found that the kind of shadowless light that you get from rows and rows of fluorescent tubes is far from satisfactory for really critical tasks. You, too, may come to prefer a strong localized light source used with lower room light. There is a very real reason for this. The sharp, definite shadows produced by such a light can be put to excellent use in determining depth and distance.

Let me give you an example. A small light source mounted close to the work table of a drill press can be adjusted to cast a sharp shadow of the drill point onto the work. As the drill is lowered, the shadow indicates just where the point will touch, and the work can be moved so that the point of the drill will meet its mark precisely. This same principle can be used in the kitchen, the office, wherever exactness counts. Watching clear shadows will aid you in many precision tasks.

Also, look into getting lights that give you a full daylight spectrum, not just *say* they do—lights that are balanced for daylight at 6500 Kelvin. If you can *see* the colors, your acuity and enjoyment of the indoor or night environment will be greatly enhanced.

However, if the full spectrum of visible light is not coming from your lamp, you cannot see colors. Remember, we see only the colors that are reflected from an object. For a demonstration go visit a quality light fixture representative—a big one in its own storefront. They will have a comparative lighting setup, and you can judge for yourself. Halogen, quartz, fluorescent, incandescent and coated light sources are all different in the wavelengths they produce.

Another small gadget that you will find invaluable in dim or dark settings is a light that goes on your key chain. This will clarify keyholes and anything else that is critical when there is no other source of light around. Putting the smallest halogen flashlight on your keys will not only come in handy, but its size will probably prevent you from losing those pesky keys ever again. A laser pointer is also of some use to guess distances in low light, because it's always the same size, can be shone around objects, and can usually penetrate fog.

Myriad gadgets and suggestions will appear on the web site as they are reviewed.

COMPUTERS

A few things are relevant to our condition in relation to computers.

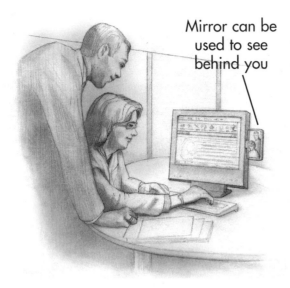

Mirror can be used to see behind you

Placing a small mirror on the monitor on your affected side will keep you informed of people moving behind you on that side.

Staring into the screen, while not damaging to your eye, can make for tension and definitely reduce blinking. You may find that using artificial tear eye drops may help eye comfort; your doctor can aid in this assessment.

Likewise, there are ways to increase the size of items on the screen. Using a larger font size will cut down on frustration and ease the placement of the cursor in the intended position. Eyestrain can make for unneeded tension. "Zoom" is almost always available under "View" in most software programs. Many writers, both monocular and binocular, use this trick.

There are also magnifiers that can increase the apparent size of a small monitor, but these are unnecessary—changing the resolution of your screen can be accomplished in a few strokes (lower resolution means larger type). So check your computer manual. You can even set this as a button so as to go between resolutions quickly.

Chapter 13

Keeping the Good Eye Good

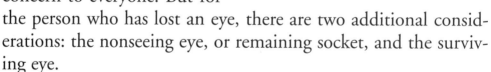

THE CARE AND safeguarding of eyesight is a matter of concern to everyone. But for the person who has lost an eye, there are two additional considerations: the nonseeing eye, or remaining socket, and the surviving eye.

What does one do about the nonseeing eye—or the eye socket, if indeed the "bad" eye has been removed? The other consideration is the overriding importance of protecting whatever eyesight remains in the surviving eye.

To get the best advice on eye care for the one-eyed, I consulted Dr. John W. McTigue, then a senior attending ophthalmologist of the Washington National Eye Center. The fruits of those interviews are contained in this chapter, on which he so generously collaborated:

1. THE EYE THAT WAS

If your damaged eye has been removed by surgery (see *enucleation, evisceration, exenteration* in the glossary), care of the remaining socket is usually very simple. When you decide on a "glass eye" or *ocular prosthesis* for cosmetic reasons, make sure it's well fitted by an expert ocularist. A poorly fitted shell can irritate the conjunctiva, the membrane that lines the eyelid and socket. This or any other irritation of the socket—from infections, foreign bodies, etc.—is usually not serious, provided you have it treated promptly by an ophthalmologist.

The socket may surprise you by continuing to perform many of the functions of a normal eye, such as cleaning itself and even shedding tears, since the lids and tear glands are usually still in working order.

If you still have your nonseeing eye, the amount of follow-up medical care it needs may vary from very frequent visits to practically none, depending on what caused the loss of vision. So make certain you understand what your condition requires in this respect. Routine follow-up care is usual in such cases.

Dr. Jerry Shields of Wills Eye Hospital adds the following:

If your nonsighted eye requires enucleation, or is already removed, a ball-shaped implant will be positioned where your eyeball was and the muscles reattached to it so that it may move. The conjunctiva is closed over it so that the implant should never appear. Thus the socket is a pouch behind the eyelids and in front of the implant—the prosthesis fits exactly into this socket and moves with the implant.

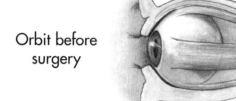

Orbit before
surgery

Enucleated orbit

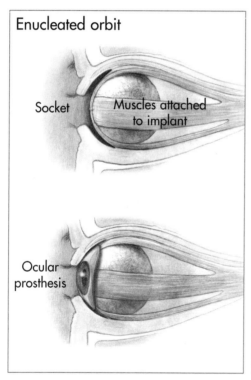

Socket

Muscles attached
to implant

Ocular
prosthesis

Exenterated orbit

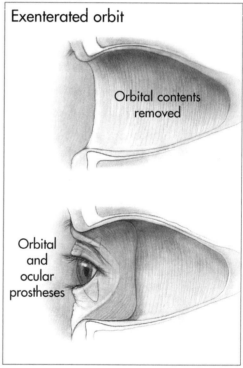

Orbital contents
removed

Orbital
and
ocular
prostheses

*The orbit before and after enucleation and exenteration.
In enucleation, the eyeball is replaced with an implant, and an
ocular prosthesis is placed above. In exenteration, the eyeball and
muscles are removed, leaving the empty socket, which is covered by
an orbital prosthesis that includes an ocular.*

2. THE GOOD EYE

Don't worry about "using up" your good eye. Your surviving eye is quite capable of taking on by itself almost all the visual tasks you need, no matter how demanding, which were once performed by both eyes together.

If your remaining eye is normal, it probably will require only routine preventive care—an ophthalmological checkup every two years may suffice. Again, be sure to consult your own doctor about this. Moreover, you should report immediately if you experience any new symptoms, such as redness, blurred vision, pain in the eye or headaches.

OTHER CONCERNS

For the one-eyed person, there are just a few special questions that relate to glasses, contact lenses and injuries or diseases of the eye.

GLASSES

Even small, subtle changes in vision can become important when you have one eye, and you'll probably be much quicker to notice them than you used to be. It may be necessary to test your eyesight for glasses more often now; some one-eyed and two-eyed patients need a test called a refraction, as frequently as every four months if their vision is changing.

Any blurring in vision may be a sign that you need new glasses. Most conditions that cause this blurring—*myopia* (nearsightedness), *hyperopia* (farsightedness), and *astigmatism* (distorted vision)—can generally be corrected by new glasses. And so can the loss of focusing power that comes with age, *presbyopia*. As the eye loses its elasticity, a bifocal or even a trifocal lens may become necessary to permit quick and easy shifts in focus.

One blessing of advancing years: The eye generally stabilizes by the age of 55 or 60. After that, you may be relatively free of vision change problems.

Once again, please be sure to use safety lenses in your glasses—your eye care professional can help.

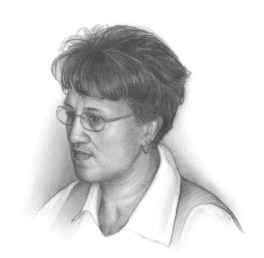

Glasses are essential to the safekeeping of your good eye.

CONTACT LENSES

For the one-eyed person who needs a corrective lens, the contact lens can be a great thing, provided that the fit is accurate, that the medical supervision is regular, and the patient is careful to exercise good sense about wearing it.

The great advantage of the contact lens is that it provides the clearest and widest visual field possible, which, of course, is of major importance to the person whose field is reduced by the loss of one eye.

In the past, with extreme cases of *myopia* or *hyperopia,* a contact lens was the only way to compensate for the loss of side vision. The situation has changed a lot with the introduction of intraocular lens implants (IOLs). This procedure is now quite standard for cataract surgery, and 90 to 95 percent or more of these patients are given IOLs. Often after these procedures, only reading glasses are necessary.

REFRACTIVE SURGERY: KERAPLASTY

New techniques for surgically changing the focusing power of the cornea are being introduced at eye centers everywhere, even advertised in the media. These are performed using advanced lasers and have proved astonishingly accurate and successful. Consult your doctor before considering this procedure.

INJURIES AND DISEASES

The person who has lost an eye must exercise special care and vigilance to prevent the development of any condition that might affect the sight of the remaining eye. Here are a few of the more common conditions.

INJURIES

No matter how trivial an injury to your remaining eye may seem to you, have your doctor examine it without delay. Only he/she can decide whether treatment is needed to ensure the safety of your remaining eye.

Should you ever be so unfortunate as to suffer a major injury to your surviving eye, don't hesitate in authorizing immediate corrective treatment. Saving any bit of vision is worth the effort required.

INFECTION

Any redness of the eye is a signal of trouble. Usually it's nothing more serious than conjunctivitis, the inflammation of the conjunctiva known as "pink eye." But don't guess at it, get prompt diagnosis and treatment. After all, it's the only one you've got.

GLAUCOMA

Your doctor can detect this insidious eye disease long before it does any damage to your vision—which is one good reason why you should never neglect your regular eye examination. Glaucoma causes damage to the optic nerve, usually through increased pressure

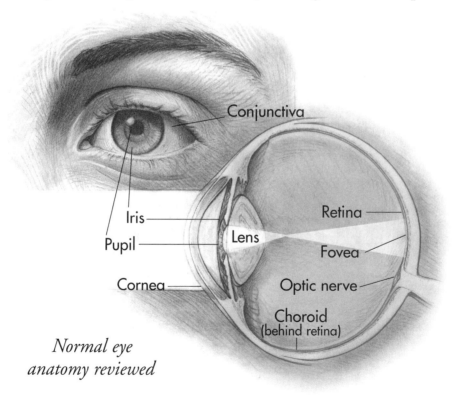

*Normal eye
anatomy reviewed*

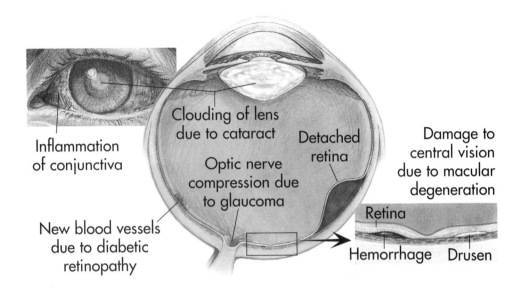

Inflammation of conjunctiva

Clouding of lens due to cataract

Optic nerve compression due to glaucoma

Detached retina

Damage to central vision due to macular degeneration

New blood vessels due to diabetic retinopathy

Retina

Hemorrhage   Drusen

Various conditions can affect the remaining eye.

within the eye. The pressure pushes on the nerve fibers and they atrophy. This increased pressure is from either too much fluid being made inside the eye or too little being drained from it.

If it's detected early, glaucoma is no cause for the one-eyed patient to despair. Prompt treatment, usually by simply using eye drops, can prevent it from doing any further damage to your vision.

CATARACT

This clouding of the lens occurs commonly among older people, even those with normal vision. When it reaches a point where it interferes significantly with normal visual activity, the natural lens can be removed by surgery. This is a procedure you can approach with every confidence that normal vision will be restored

.

DETACHED RETINA

The retina has fallen away from its normal position in the back of the eye. It's just as if the film is no longer in the right position—vision is affected because the receptors are displaced. Symptoms include flashing lights, floating blurry objects, and/or a moving "curtain" over your field of vision. You need to see your ophthalmologist immediately if any of these symptoms occur. The retina can be repositioned by surgery or by a laser, usually returning the patient's previous vision.

The *retina* is actually mostly attached to the back of the normal eye by an active pumping function of the *choroid* beneath it. Detachments can be due to a tiny retinal hole, effectively losing the "seal" of the "pump". Detachments often heal after the hole is sealed down again to restore the retina's position and protect vision. If a detachment is longstanding, the retina loses nutrition and can be damaged.

DIABETES

If you are diagnosed as having diabetes, special attention should be paid by your ophthalmologist toward noting any changes in the eye. Diabetic retinopathy cannot be detected by you, though your eye doctor can see it in the back of your eye. Often it's best to get special photographs of the back of your eye so that any change can be compared at the next exam. Diabetic patients will need to make regular appointments with the eye doctor their first priority because the condition can produce new blood vessels that can threaten eyesight and detach the retina if untreated.

Other, rarer diseases that affect the eye are treatable—especially if detected early—so do not miss your eye exams. And take notice of *any* changes, such as pain when you brush the hair on your temples. These need to be reported to your doctor, so write them down. For all its apparent

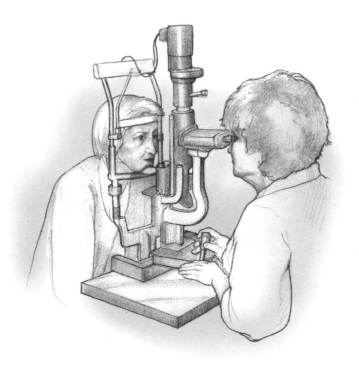

Regular eye exams are a must.

delicacy, the eye is a tough and resilient organ and really requires only a little care. Since you only have the one, take care of yourself.

Agencies that deal with the preservation of sight are constantly warning of eye hazards, and the one-eyed would do well to pay attention. The Prevent Blindness America is one leading organization and is linked at the web site, as is The National Federation of the Blind and others. Every state has an office. Other resource agencies are listed as well, and their addresses updated.

Low vision in the surviving eye is treated no differently than low vision for binocular people, given that one-eyed individuals can get low-vision aids and prescriptions in their protective glasses.

Chapter 14

Seeing to Your Looks

IN MOST CASES, the simple loss of vision on one side has no effect whatsoever on the appearance, and it's visually difficult for another person to tell which is the "working" eye. If you've suffered more severe injury, however, and the eye has been surgically removed, or if further damage to the surrounding tissues is evident, you will have some—hopefully temporary—problems with the way you look.

Today, ophthalmic plastic surgery and custom fitting of an ocular prosthesis by an ocularist can minimize or eliminate any evidence of imbalance between the two eyes. That said, your situation may differ. More extensive surgery on the orbit, or plastic surgery on the socket and eyelids can bring your appearance closer to normal. Time will tell. Everyone is different.

If a damaged eye remains, or if the prosthesis is ill-fitting, there may be some change in appearance caused by the two pupils not tracking precisely in unison. In other words, it may look like you are seeing in two directions: The eyes may seem perfectly aligned when looking straight ahead, but diverge a bit when the good eye glances to one side. While head movement minimizes this, the effect is usually not all that displeasing. Often the ocularist can disguise an unsightly or deviating eye under a thin scleral shell prosthesis.

In fact, many of us are intrigued by a slight cast in a pleasant face—it seems to add a certain individuality. Indeed, as Patrick Trevor-Roper notes in his book *The World Through Blunted Sight,* earlier societies considered a "squint" (difference in the direction of the eyes) a sign of godliness and beauty. He reminds us that many a great artist has gone so far as to paint their portrait subjects with an exaggerated divergence of the eyes, more white showing in the eye closest to the viewer.

What makes these observations so important is that the way you look may not be nearly as important as the way you *think* you look to others.

Tips from your ocularist will help you look your individual best while talking and moving about in the world.

We all know people who become so uncomfortable under the direct gaze of another person that they look away. This natural shyness can become exaggerated for anyone who is unsure of their appearance. A determined effort to look people straight in the eye is perhaps the best way to overcome this self-consciousness! While this may seem foreign to you right now, you can consciously change the way you appear in this manner. What you may consider to be brash boldness here will make a huge difference in your confidence. As a matter of fact, looking away may only emphasize a perceived problem. Look 'em straight in the eye, even when you don't want to, and you'll be surprised at the reaction. A direct gaze is assumed to be confident and out-going because people will think you are more interested in *them*.

Annie N. is 18 years old. "When people spoke to me, I looked away, probably thinking that if I couldn't see their eyes, they couldn't see mine. More than once, I was accused of being rude— not interested in what the other person had to say. I still sometimes look away, but I now know why, and so I try hard to focus."

"Most important," says Sue Moran, the TV personality mentioned in Chapter 11, "is to look at things and people straight-on, turning or raising the head, not just the eyes. That's especially important when looking up at someone from, say, a seated position."

Mrs. Moran also has a word of advice to women who may be concerned about the "bright" look of an artificial eye. "You can do a lot with make-up, especially with eye shadow, to make your eyes look more alike. False eyelashes have been very useful." Today, these don't have to look exaggerated. "They add shadows and soften the 'starry' look you sometimes see with a prosthesis."

Sandy Duncan, the actress, also makes good use of false eyelashes. In a magazine interview, she described with great sense of humor how difficult it was at first to affix the strip to her good eye, which must be kept closed during the process. She once wore fashionably tinted glasses as a presenter at the Academy Awards. Though these fashions come and go, the tint helped her mask the slight difference in how her eyes moved.

Teresa W. is monocular and a prosthetic eye wearer. Not only is she a cosmetics salesperson, but very successful. She has embraced her loss and never lets it discourage her. She has a terrifically positive attitude and has developed many tricks in applying eye makeup.

Lizanne Johnson, an ocularist, has offered many techniques

for making the eyes not only look alike, but specifics on great illusions in make-up for monocular women. One definitive tip she relates is that in working with eye shadow. The use of light shadow generally makes an illusion of more room, while dark shadow gives the illusion of less room. This can be adapted for a smaller eye, *ptosis,* or superior sulcus.

Different types of make-up relate to different individuals—like the differences among eyeliners used for various eye shapes and eyelids.

WITHOUT MAKE-UP

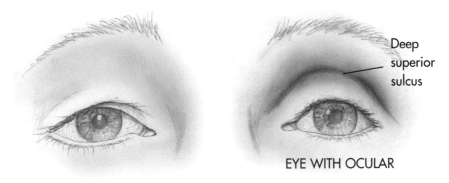

WITH MAKE-UP MODIFICATIONS

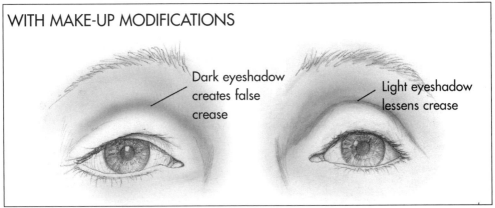

Using eyeshadow can even out any differences in the look of your eyes. Here, disguising a deeper superior sulcus.

In earlier male fashions, the black eyepatch seemed to be a symbol not of loss but of achievement. It endowed movie stars and military men with charisma, even becoming a trademark for some, like General Moshe Dayan of Israel.

As a matter of fact, the actor John Wayne didn't win an Oscar until he appeared in an eyepatch! For now the eyepatch seems dated, but it may have a comeback sooner than later. One rock star already seems to be bringing it back as a sign of virility, and several animated characters make use of it as a sign of toughness and perseverance.

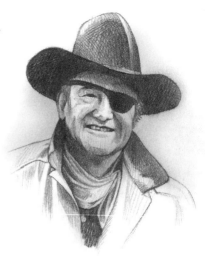

Actor John Wayne

Chapter 15

Eye-making (Ocularistry)

WHILE NOT EVERYONE who reads this book wears an artificial eye (ocular prosthesis), a significant number do, which warrants greater detail on this unique and interesting craft.

Except in fairly unusual situations, anyone whose eye has been removed can expect to wear an artificial eye called a *prosthesis*. Your ophthalmologist normally will recommend that a trained ocularist do the fitting, and that you have a custom prosthesis made. Most larger cities have at least one ocularist to serve the population's needs.

The artificial eye, as we know it today, has a long history. While the inventor of the artificial eye is difficult to trace, clearly they were being used by the time of Shakespeare. Just before then, Ambroise Pare', the father of surgery, was one of the

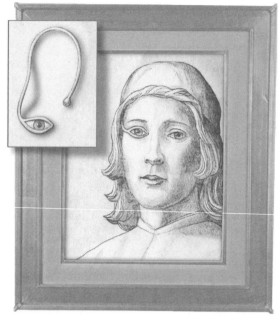

Renaissance youth wearing a ekblepharon eye prosthesis, worn over the eyelid.

first to describe the use of an artificial eye to fit over the eyelids. These were made of gold and silver. These were known as ekblepharon eye prostheses. The Venetians were noted as developing the first ocular prosthesis to be worn over a shrunken eye, behind the eyelids, since enucleation only became standard practice in the early 1800s.

Enamel prostheses were attractive, but expensive and not durable. German craftsmen in 1835 are credited with the first definitive cryolite glass eyes, using colored glass to imitate the natural color of the iris. Later in the 19th century, German eye craftsmen began touring the U.S. and fitting artificial eyes to patients. Stock eyes were also fitted from the drawer, using simply "best fit."

Today's plastic human eyes (ocular prostheses) evolved in the United States during the years surrounding World War II with the development of polymethylmethacrylate and have since become the standard. These impressions fit prosthetic eyes are now molded to fit the socket over the implant, thus allowing for the greatest range of motion. With the proper professional fit and fabrication, the socket virtually cleans itself, and these eyes are long lasting and a beautiful match.

In the case of more extensive tissue damage surrounding the eye and eyelids, an external prosthesis can be fashioned by an ocularist or an anaplastologist, a professional who specializes in facial prostheses using silicone. This is generally affixed to the face by adhesives or attaching it to implants. The improvement that these prostheses generate can be alarmingly lifelike. The refinement of ocular implants and surgical procedures have greatly improved the end results these professionals can achieve. Sometimes even trained observers miss detecting an artificial eye—and I myself have been fooled! Once an ocularist asked after someone left the office, "How did you like my work?" "On whom?" I said, thinking that surely I could tell. The ocularist had trained his patient well to move her head instead of her eyes, and chuckled with glee at my confusion, though I had spoken directly with her not two feet away.

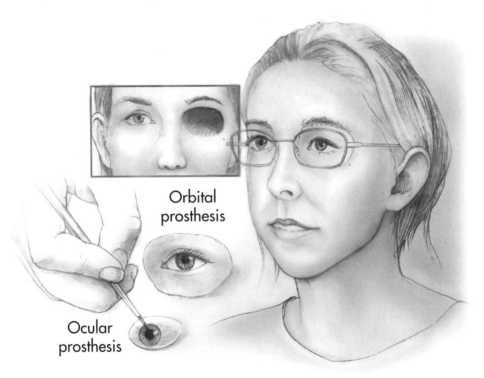

Orbital
prosthesis

Ocular
prosthesis

An ocular prosthesis replaces a lost eye, while an orbital prosthesis goes over an empty socket, replacing both the eye and eyelids. Both prostheses are custom-made for the patient.

Chapter 16

Driving and Piloting Licenses

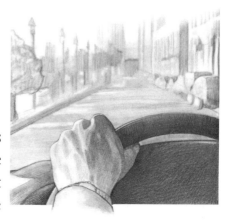

"**W**ILL I BE allowed to drive?"

That is one of the first questions likely to come to the mind of the newly monocular. The fact is that regulations vary from state to state in the U.S., so there's no one answer.

However, much has been done in recent years to bring state regulations into line with nationally recommended vision standards for drivers, and today all 50 states as well as the District of Columbia license one-eyed drivers who pass their visual tests. These regulations also change, so you can get all the current information at the web site. That is the best way for us to keep you up to date.

In a jointly published booklet on visual screening for driver licensing, The American Association of Motor Vehicle

Administrators and the American Optometric Association remark that "most drivers are anxious to retain driving privileges and as a result they learn to compensate for deficiencies."

As to flying regulations, once a licensed pilot loses an eye, the medical certificate is revoked for a period of adaptation, usually about six months. Then, after an eye exam, the information is examined by the FAA, and a student license is issued, followed by an adaptation period and an FAA exam. With satisfactory performance the former certificate is reissued. A recent count showed 218 first, 739 second, and 2,623 thirdclass medical certificates issued to monocular pilots! Monocularity *is* compatible with the flying you once enjoyed.

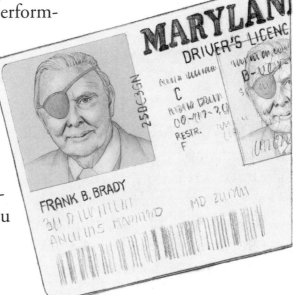

Driving and other vehicle licenses are affected,
though there are ways to proceed.

Chapter 17

For Parents Only

WHAT CAN PARENTS tell a child who has just lost an eye? If they haven't had the same experience, can they truly relate to what their loved one is experiencing? Can they even talk about it?

In any case, parents should, of course, approach the topic with sensitivity, since the child's emotional outlook is the biggest effect of eye loss—it can be greater than the physical loss and last just as long.

To get a better understanding of the problem, I talked with parents, pediatric ophthalmologists, child psychiatrists, persons who had lost an eye as a child, and the children themselves who had just lost vision in one eye.

Dr. Nancy Mansfield (director, Social Services, Childrens Hospital, Los Angeles) notes: "The grief parents experience when it is their child who has lost the vision of an eye or lost the eye itself is different than the grief that the child experiences."

There seems to be general agreement on several points. Discussions of the loss must be adjusted according to the child's age, emotional stability, maturity, natural coordination, athletic inclination and the child-parent relationship. Moreover, if the parents rec-

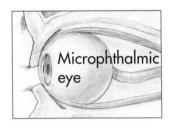
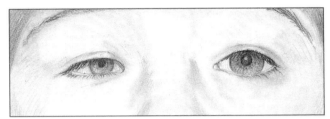
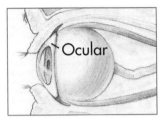
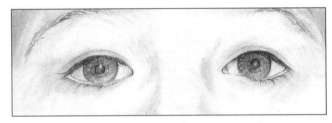

The underdeveloped microphthalmic eye can be corrected using a scleral cover shell ocular prosthesis.

ognize the true impact of eye loss, this will help them maintain a calm, dispassionate attitude that can prevent the buildup of exaggerated fears. Certainly, emotional displays in the presence of the child are out of order. Experts all agree that children, in general, adapt quickly, and that the younger the child (especially if born blind in one eye), the quicker and more complete is the adaptation.

Aileen H. related the story of her beautiful daughter, Elizabeth.

"She was born micropthalmic, which means her right eye never fully developed. Elizabeth wears a prosthesis and protective glasses, but not many people even realize that she is blind on that side. If there is a disadvantage, she never knew what she was missing by having just one eye. She is bright and cheerful, never using it as an excuse for anything, and she never complains. Her father and I have never tried to limit her activities.

However there was one instance where another parent commented, and we were both shocked. It was soccer season. As you know, soccer at age five looks more like herding sheep. Several of the girls on the field were milling about, seemingly lost or disinterested. When we decided to switch her from soccer to swimming, one mother (who knew of Elizabeth's condition) said, 'Oh, I understand—the eye problem must have been an obstacle!'

'No,' we replied, 'her vision had nothing to do with it. She just hates soccer!' She went on to the all-stars that summer swimming season with the fastest times in her age group. We were both surprised that this particular mother thought Elizabeth was leaving soccer because of a percieved disability instead of her lack of interest in soccer!"

Parents who tend to be overprotective can learn from this and the example of the late Morris Udall, congressman from Arizona and a presidential candidate in 1976. When I met him in his Capitol Hill office, he spoke of his own experience.

"At the age of six, I suffered a serious injury to my right eye, which eventually led to surgery to remove the eye. The loss of the eye, however, never interfered with my ability or opportunity to engage in athletic events in high school, college or as a professional. I can also state unequivocally that the wearing of a glass eye never lead to, nor contributed to, any injury in athletic competition.

In high school in St. James, Arizona, I played quarterback on the football team and was captain of the basketball team. While at the University of Arizona, I played three years of varsity basketball and even led the team in scoring one of those years. In fact, my shooting ability was good enough to bring an allegation by a rival fan that 'Udall can't shoot that well with only one eye!'

Although my college career was interrupted by service in the Army Air Corps during World War II, I continued to play basketball and organized a team, which was, in part, made up of one-eyed players.

After college, I played a year of professional basketball with the Denver Nuggets of the NBL.

In addition, I obtained a private pilot's license and have logged over 4,000 hours of flight time.

While my career has been in law and public service, in my opinion the loss of my eye did not nor would not have interfered with my ability to compete professionally in athletics."

Whenever parents asked, he would write letters to children who had lost vision in one eye to reassure them. Udall credited his mother for "doing all the right things" following the accident. She never restricted his activities. She allowed him to play normally and engage in sports. When I asked "Mo" if his drive to overcome his disadvantage played a role in his achievements, he said he was determined as a youngster that he could do anything as well as anyone else could, or better. He believed that his loss pushed him further than he otherwise would have gone.

I've appeared on occasion as an expert witness in court cases regarding vision loss. I believe that every effort should be made to safeguard the child's psyche and weigh that against any settlement, and that parents should be willing to let it go if the risk to the child is too great.

A final point: Kids can be cruel about physical traits that differentiate one from the group. A one-eyed child is likely to be the subject of these attacks, particularly if his condition is noticed by special attention, bandages, special glasses, etc.

Annie N. wrote,

> "My friends ask me what it's like seeing out of one eye. Since I was born this way, I can't easily relate the difference between my vision and theirs. So sometimes I ask them to tape one eye shut and then go about their day. Before long they get frustrated, particularly after they've toppled down a staircase or misjudged the height of a curb. They quickly pull off the tape, and their full vision is restored!
>
> For 18 years, I wanted to take off the tape too, but I couldn't.
>
> It wasn't until I was mainstreamed in a regular kindergarten classroom that I became aware that my eyes were 'different.' Now I had to explain why one eye tended to stay closed. I was accused of cheating when I only covered my sighted eye for hide and seek, and I would be the last chosen for PE. Some adults would ask my mother—right in front of me as if I weren't there or was deaf—what was wrong with my eyes. Living with one eye all my life has certainly made me a stronger person."

Since it's impractical to isolate the child, some advance counseling is a good idea. If she or he has self-confidence, the one-eyed youth might just laugh it off, but not all children are able to do this. As long as children know that losing one eye does not limit their potential, self-esteem can grow. Let them know, too, that they are in great company.

Chapter 18

Senior Class

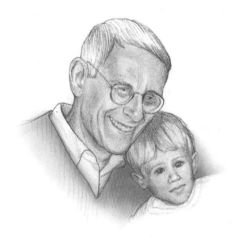

LOSS OF VISION in one eye is not a trivial thing at any age, but the problems of adjusting to the loss can become more critical to a person of advanced years. Slowed reaction times, less than perfect vision in the remaining eye, deterioration of hearing (a sense that often supplements sight) are all among the negative factors. On the positive side, however, are experience, judgment and skill built up over the years. These traits, both positive and negative, tend to balance out and allow the older segment of the population to compare favorably with the automobile safety record of the somewhat-more-accident-prone young drivers.

One of the greatest concerns of older people is the thought of giving up their driving privileges because of vision limitations (some states only license monoculars for daytime). A lifetime of

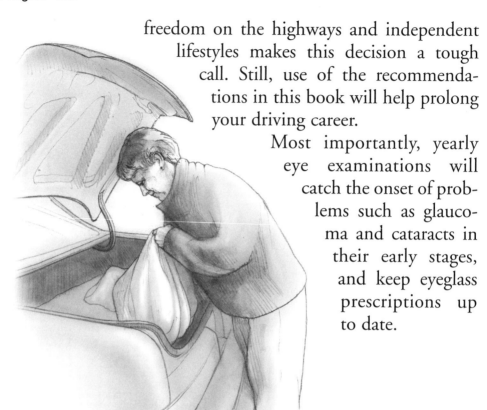

freedom on the highways and independent lifestyles makes this decision a tough call. Still, use of the recommendations in this book will help prolong your driving career.

Most importantly, yearly eye examinations will catch the onset of problems such as glaucoma and cataracts in their early stages, and keep eyeglass prescriptions up to date.

Loss of an eye does not have to represent loss of independence among senior citizens.

Chapter 19

Great Company

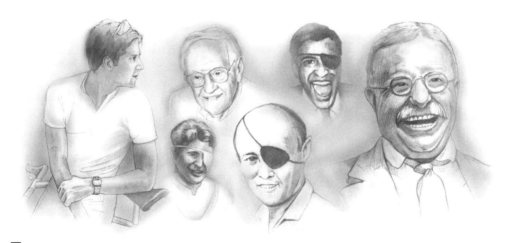

THROUGHOUT HISTORY PEOPLE with all kinds of obstacles have distinguished themselves in all walks of life, and in this book I've cited the accomplishments of just some public figures, entertainers, scientists, pilots, and athletes who have overcome the problem and inconvenience of one-eyed sight. For the person who has just joined this club, it may be interesting and encouraging to note a few of its more prominent members and the diversity of their accomplishments. We may be adding your name to this list soon!

Theodore Roosevelt, the vigorous U.S. President who, while in office, lost his left eye in a boxing bout with a naval officer.

Moshe Dayan, Israeli military leader and statesman. A World War II gunfire accident took his left eye but didn't dampen a distinguished pubic career.

Ian Smith, prime minister of Rhodesia, center of worldwide controversy.

Morris K. Udall, congressman and 1976 candidate for Presidential nomination, who lost his right eye at age six, but didn't let that keep him from scholastic and professional athletics, flying, and public service.

Sammy Davis, Jr., the irrepressible entertainer who didn't achieve superstardom until after an automobile accident cost him the sight of his left eye.

John Ford, top movie director.

Peter Falk, plodding star of the long-running TV series "Columbo," who solves crimes with one eye.

Hilaire Germain Edgar Degas, master French impressionist who did some of his finest work after he lost his right eye in the siege of Paris.

John Milton, 17th-century poet.

Julius Axelrod, 1970 Nobel Prize winner in physiology and medicine, whose graduate work and Nobel Prize efforts came from a laboratory accident in which he lost his left eye.

Guglielmo Marconi, inventor of the radio.

Wiley Post, pioneering aviator who, with vision only in his right eye, made the first solo circumnavigation of the globe in seven days, 18 hours, 49 minutes. Post made many contributions to

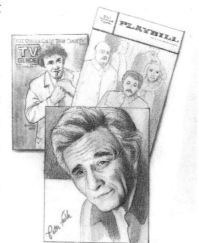

Monocular actor Peter Falk has had a great, lengthy career.

flight technology.

Pierce Holt, aggressive defensive tackle for the Forty-Niners played in Superbowl XXIII and again in Superbowl XXIV with only 10 percent vision in his left eye.

Elizabeth Blackwell, the first woman to graduate from an American medical school (1849) lost an eye while in postgraduate school in France.

Hannibal became practically one-eyed from an infection while making his legendary crossing of the Alps in 218 B.C.

Losing an eye will not guarantee greatness, but there is nothing about it that means you are limited. "Go, and do thou likewise." Chances are, you will be more aware of your surroundings than your two-eyed companions.

One story of such a feat is that of Admiral Nelson, one of the greatest of British naval heroes, whose victory at Trafalgar occurred more than ten years after he lost his right eye in a battle off Corsica. Nelson even used his blind eye to advantage in the historic Battle of Copenhagen in 1801. His superior, Sir Hyde Parker, had signaled him to halt his attack on a Danish ship against what Parker considered very doubtful odds. Nelson purposefully placed a telescope against his blind eye, and after a careful "look," told his aide. "I do not see the signal." He then proceeded with the attack, which was soon to become a major chapter in Britain's proud naval history. Thus Nelson used his handicap to turn a potential defeat into a resounding victory.

What might you add to this list? Almost anything!

Your world awaits!

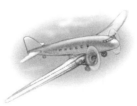

Glossary

Accommodation: Adjustments made to focus on objects nearby, including lens thickening, pupil constriction

Aqueous humor: Watery fluid inside the front of the eye

Affected side: The side toward your visual loss

Amblyopia: Visual loss typically in one eye, due to a defect in image processing by the brain

AMD: Age-related macular degeneration

Amsler grid: A test for macular degeneration and macular function

Anaplastologist: A professional who restores (through prosthetic means) a malformed or absent part of the human body, including orbitals (eye and surrounding anatomy)

Anatomy: Having to do with naming parts of the body

Anophthalmos, *Anophthalmic:* A developmental defect characterized by complete absence of the eye

Anterior chamber: The fluid-filled space between the iris/lens and the inside of the cornea

Apparent size: The relative amount of space an object occupies in the visual field

Artificial eye: A custom-made plastic duplicate of your other eye; see ocular prosthesis

Astigmatism: Distorted vision due to corneal or lenticular irregularity or shape

Binocularity, binocular: Having or using two eyes, which gives the brain information to make a picture of the world in space; see monocular

Blind spot: A defect in the field of vision—one at the optic nerve is normal

Blur Interpretation: The ability to discriminate and identify an unclear image of an object by relying on context, color and overall shape cues

Cataract: Clouding of the lens behind the iris causing blurry vision; this can occur from injury or disease or aging

Choroid: The vascular layer behind the retina, in front of the sclera

Congenital: From birth; anything you were born with

Conjunctiva: Thin layer of tissue lining the inside of the lids, continues onto the sclera, or lining the socket

Conjunctival sac: The socket

Contrast: The difference between light and shadow or various colors

Convergence: The eyes look together at objects nearby

Cornea: The outermost, front-most clear layer of the eye; does most of the focusing of images onto the retina

Cosmesis: For the benefit of appearance, looks

Critical distance: Farthest point from which an object can be visually discriminated

Critical feature: The parts of an object that yield the most information

Depth: The relative distance of objects and their spatial relationship to each other

Diabetes: Disease affecting the pancreas and the blood sugar

Diabetic retinopathy: Sight-threatening changes in the retina due to diabetes

Diagnosis: Naming the disease of a patient

Dilation, iris: Opening of the iris wider, making the pupil larger

Dimension, 2-D: A two-dimensional view is flat like a photograph

Dimension, 3-D: A three-dimensional view that has spatial depth

Discrimination: The ability to make distinctions within and/or between visible things

Disparity: Difference between two images or the motion of two things

Distance: An interval between two points in space or time

Ectropion: Turning out of the eyelashes

Entropion: Turning in of the eyelashes

Enophthalmos: Sinking inwards of the eye

Enucleation: Surgical removal of the eyeball

Epithelium: The outermost cell layer of any tissue

Evisceration: Surgical removal of only the inside of the eye, leaving the sclera

Exenteration: Surgical removal of most of the tissues in the orbit

Extraocular muscles: Muscles outside of the eyeball that move the eye

Exophthalmos: Bulging outwards of the eye

Extrude, extrusion: Pushed out, sometimes showing the implant surface

Eye-hand/body coordination: Use of vision to direct body movements more efficiently and easily

Familiar size: The typical size of any object based upon the individual's learning experience

Farsightedness: A visual disorder whereby an image entering the visual system (the eye) lands behind the retina causing vision to be clearer at distances than up close

Fixation: Maintaining eye position and focusing gaze on a target

Fornix (plural is fornices): The corner of the conjunctival sac or socket

Fovea: The center of the macula, used for finest vision

Fusion: The melding of two images into a single 3-D picture

Glass eye: An ocular prosthesis, usually made of plastic

Glaucoma: Disease causing nerve damage to the optic nerve, usually by too much pressure in the eyeball

Glaucoma, congenital: Glaucoma caused by blockage of the outflow of the aqueous humor, usually from birth

Glaucoma, low pressure: Caused by high sensitivity to pressure

Hemangioma: A tumor, usually harmless, made up of blood vessels

Hyperopia: See farsightedness

Hydroxyapatite: An ocular implant made from sterilized coral

Implant: Any object sutured into the body. In enucleation, a ball that takes the place of the eyeball—the extraocular muscles are attached to make the implant move with the other eye, covered by the conjunctival sac.

Impression: A casting of the tissues around the socket used to make a custom prosthesis

Infection: An invasion of the body typically caused by bacteria or viruses

Inferior: Toward the bottom

Inflammation: Redness of tissues from the body's protective reaction to irritation, inury or infection by bringing more blood to the area

Intraocular: Inside the eyeball

Interposition: Visual cue that enables comparative distance judgment (i.e., closer vs. farther away). When one object is in front of and partially blocks another, the object being blocked is farther away. The object fully seen is closer to the observer.

Iris: The colored part of the eye that regulates the amount of light coming into the retina; located behind the cornea, in front of the lens

Keratopathy: Any disease of the cornea

Laser: A powerful light that heats up or destroys tissue, usually in surgery

Lasik surgery: One type of refractive keratoplasty performed with a laser

Lens: The element of the eye that finely focuses the light into an image

Localization: Visually finding a target

Low vision: Lower than normal vision, often gradual

Macula: Sensitive area of the retina responsible for central vision

Macular degeneration: Breakdown of the macula causing central loss of vision

Malignant: Cancerous, spreading tumor

Medpor©: Synthetic, porous ocular implant

Melanoma: Cancerous tumor from cells that contain pigment (melanin)

Migration: Moving from where intended

Microphthalmia: Congenital disease in which the eyeball never fully developed

Monocular: Referring to having or using only one eye

Motility: Movement of the eye by muscles

Motion disparity: Difference in the moving of two or more objects

Movement: Change in position of part or all of an object

Myopia: A visual disorder whereby an image entering the visual system lands in front of the retina, causing vision to be clearer up close than at distances. Also called Nearsightedness

Nearsightedness: See Myopia

Nerve: A 'cable' carrying electrical signals to or from the brain

Object: Any visible form, person, picture or substance in the environment

Ocularist: Trained professional who fits and makes ocular prosthetics or artificial eyes

Ocular: Pertaining to the eye

Ocular prosthesis: An artificial eye

Oculoplastic: Medical specialty to perform plastic surgery near the eyes

OD: Pertaining to the right eye (oculus dexter); OS is left

Ophthalmologist: Medical doctor specializing in the diseases and treatment of the eye

Optic nerve: Large nerve that carries signals to the brain from the retina

Optician: Eye care professional who fits and makes glasses

Optimum viewing angle: That angle which provides maximum visibility and minimum discomfort while looking at an object

Optometrist (O.D.): Medical professional specializing in the eye with the exception of performing surgery

Orbit: The bony cone in the skull surrounding the eyeball, nerves and muscles

Orbital prosthesis: Device that replaces both the eye and the orbital contents

OS: Pertaining to the left eye (os sinister); OD is right

Palpebral fissure: The opening between the eyelids

Pathology: The study of diseases; anything wrong with the body

Peripheral vision: Outer region of the visual field

Periphery: Outermost part

Perspective: One of several ways to tell distance on a two-dimensional plane

Perspective, atmospheric: Objects in front are sharper than those in the distance

Perspective, contrast: Colors, distinct shadows and highlights lessen with distance

Perspective, overlap: Objects in front cross over and cover our view of objects behind

Perspective, vanishing: Objects get smaller and closer together in the distance

Posterior: Part toward the back

Preferred viewing distance: Distance at which an object can be most easily discriminated and/or correctly identified

Presbyopia: With age, the flexibility of the lens of the eye is less, causing images to blur up close

Prognosis: The most likely future of a patient

Prosthesis: Artificial eye; anything that replaces normal anatomy

Ptosis: Droopy eyelid

Ptisis bulbi: Eyeball that is shrunken, scarred

Pupil: Hole in the iris allowing light to the retina, gets larger in dilation, smaller in constriction

Refractive keratoplasty: Surgery to correct vision by reshaping the cornea

Relative movement: Moving your eye/head/body in order to appreciate an object's location (in space)

Retina, retinal: Light-sensitive part of the eye, like the film in a camera; referring to the retina

Retinitis pigmentosa: Progressively blinding disease affecting the pigment in the eye

Retinoblastoma: Congenital tumor inside the eye

Retinopathy, diabetic: Either nonproliferative leaking of the blood vessels in the retina or proliferative fibrosis and new vessels on the retina due to complications of diabetes

Retinopathy, proliferative: Diabetic retinopathy possibly causing retinal detachment

Retinopathy, sympathetic: The good eye is threatened to catch the disease of the damaged eye

Scanning: Use of eye and head movements to search for a target

Sclera: White, tough outer coating of the eyeball

Scleral shell: A type of thin prosthesis worn over a nonseeing eye

Socket: The conjunctival sac in front of the implant that holds an artificial eye

Spatial relationships: The ability to orient one's body in space and to perceive the position of objects in relation to oneself and to other objects

Square off: Use of one's body for establishing a perpendicular alignment to a straight surface

Stereopsis: The ability to use three-dimensional binocular vision

Sulcus; superior sulcus: Deep skin groove around the upper eyelid; "superior sulcus" means a hollow above the upper eyelid

Superior: Toward the top

Sympathetic ophthalmia: Disease of the sightless eye affecting the good eye

Tactual: The sense of touch

Target: A visual object, symbol or event in the environment

Tears, artificial: Moistening eye drops

Three-dimensional (3-D) form perception: The ability to identify tangible concrete objects

Tonometry: Test of the pressure inside the eye

Topography: Physical features of a place or region

Tracing: Visually following a stationary line

Tracking: Visually following a moving object

Two-dimensional (2-D) form perception: The ability to identify pictures of objects, such as photographs or directions on environmental signs

Visual acuity: Strength of vision; example: A visual acuity (VA) of 20/20 is seeing at 20 feet what a normal eye sees at 20 feet; 20/200 is seeing at 20 feet what a normal eye sees at 200 feet, thus worse vision

Visual closure: Identifying a target when only part of it can be seen

Visual field: Test of the range of vision side to side, up to down

Vitreous, vitrectomy: Posterior fluid in the eyeball

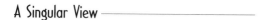

See the web site **www.asingularview.com** for information and updates on tips, products and techniques. This is the best way to get current information because changing the site is much easier than sending you a new book!

You are a special invited guest at the site, now that you have this book.